74.00

MEDICAL
INTELLIGENCE
UNIT

REDUCED-SIZE LUNG TRANSPLANTATION

John A. Kern, M.D.
Irving L. Kron, M.D.
University of Virginia

R.G. LANDES COMPANY
AUSTIN

MEDICAL INTELLIGENCE UNIT

REDUCED-SIZE LUNG TRANSPLANTATION

R.G. LANDES COMPANY
Austin / Georgetown

CRC Press is the exclusive worldwide distributor of publications of the Medical Intelligence Unit.
CRC Press, 2000 Corporate Blvd. NW, Boca Raton, FL 33431. Phone: 407/994-0555.

Submitted: April 1993
Published: June 1993

Production: Carol Harwell
Copy Editor: Constance Kerkaporta

Please address all inquiries to the Publisher:
R.G. Landes Company
909 Pine Street
Georgetown, TX 78626
or
P.O. Box 4858
Austin, TX 78765
Phone: 512/ 863 7762
FAX: 512/ 863 0081

ISBN 1-879702-69-X
CATALOG # LN-0269

CONTRIBUTORS

William A. Baumgartner, M.D.
Division of Cardiac Surgery
The Johns Hopkins Medical Institutions
Baltimore, Maryland

Charles D. Fraser, Jr., M.D.
Division of Cardiac Surgery
The Johns Hopkins Medical Institutions
Baltimore, Maryland

Charles B. Huddleston, M.D.
Division of Cardiothoracic Surgery
Department of Surgery
Washington University
School of Medicine
St. Louis, Missouri

John A. Kern, M.D.
Division of Cardiothoracic Surgery
Department of Surgery
The University of Virginia
    Health Sciences Center
Charlottesville, Virginia

Irving L. Kron, M.D.
Division of Cardiothoracic Surgery
Department of Surgery
The University of Virginia
    Health Sciences Center
Charlottesville, Virginia

Scott E. Langenburg, M.D.
Department of Surgery
The University of Virginia
    Health Sciences Center
Charlottesville, Virginia

Douglas K. Martin, B.Sc.
Centre for Bioethics
University of Toronto
Toronto, Ontario

Mark Siegler, M.D.
Center for Clinical Medical Ethics
Department of Medicine
The University of Chicago Pritzker
    School of Medicine
Chicago, Illinois

Peter A. Singer, M.D., M.P.H.,
    F.R.C.P., F.A.C.P.
Centre for Bioethics
Department of Medicine
University of Toronto
Toronto, Ontario

Thomas L. Spray, M.D.
Division of Cardiothoracic Surgery
Department of Surgery
Washington University
School of Medicine
St. Louis, Missouri

Vaughn A. Starnes, M.D.
Division of Cardiothoracic Surgery
Childrens Hospital Los Angeles
University of Southern California
Los Angeles, California

Pierre R. Theodore, B.A.
Division of Cardiothoracic Surgery
Childrens Hospital Los Angeles
University of Southern California
Los Angeles, California

Curtis G. Tribble, M.D.
Division of Cardiothoracic Surgery
Department of Surgery
The University of Virginia Health
    Sciences Center
Charlottesville, Virginia

PREFACE

This book describes research and clinical issues relavant to reduced-size lung transplantation. Topics include clinical and investigative issues unique to this specialized discipline. Current thoughts on pulmonary preservation, the technique of experimental reduced-size lung transplantation and the ethical considerations of living related donor lung transplantation are reviewed.

The pediatric patient with end-stage lung disease has two donor options: size matched immature whole lungs or reduced-size mature lobes. The pool of donors of immature whole lungs is small. This fact makes reduced-size lung transplantation particularly appealing. The advent of reduced-size lung transplantation has set the stage for this new frontier in lung transplantation. We hope that this monograph will serve as a valuable guide for the generation of new questions and continued exploration in this most interesting area of work.

CONTENTS

ACKNOWLEDGMENT

The editors wish to thank the contributors to this book for their timely contributions and excellent reviews. In addition, we would like to thank the publisher for giving us the opportunity to collect this information for others to review.

CHAPTER 1

INTRODUCTION

Irving L. Kron
Curtis G. Tribble
John A. Kern

The modern era of lung transplantation began with the Toronto group's first successful single lung transplant in 1983.[1] Previous efforts at lung transplantation failed due to problems with airway healing and the inability to adequately prevent rejection. In the early 1980s Cooper and his colleagues developed the concept of the omental wrap to aid bronchial anastomotic healing.[2] This technique along with the introduction of improved immuno-suppressive drugs helped usher in the successful era of lung transplantation. The growth of the discipline of lung transplantation has been rapid but at the same time limited by a severe shortage of donor organs. Part of the organ shortage problem is the difficulty in optimally matching donors with recipients. In addition, growing indications for single and double lung transplantation are placing an even greater demand on the already limited donor lung pool.

Simultaneous heart-lung transplantation has been required less frequently because of the ability to repair many intracardiac defects at the time of double lung transplantation when the indication for lung replacement is pulmonary hypertension. In addition, it has recently been noted that single lung transplantation is also possible for emphysema and other noninfective lung diseases previously believed to be inappropriately treated through single lung replacement. Finally, age limits for lung transplant recipients have broadened now that pediatric lung transplantation is more commonly practiced.[3] For all of these reasons there are not enough transplantable lungs available to meet the current demand.

The most important issue limiting more widespread practice of lung transplantation is the relative lack of suitable lung donors. It has been

Reduced-size Lung Transplantation, edited by John A. Kern, M.D. and Irving L. Kron, M.D.; © 1993 R.G. Landes Company.

estimated that only one in ten acceptable cardiac donors is also an acceptable lung donor. This has resulted in mortality on lung waiting lists to be as high as 50%. One reason for this is that lung donation criteria in the past have been strict. These criteria have included adequate oxygenation with a PO_2 greater than 400 mmHg on 100% FIO_2, lack of purulent secretions by bronchoscopy, lack of infiltrates on chest radiograph, lack of lung or airway injury as well as a relatively stable donor less than fifty-five years of age.[4] We have recently demonstrated that these criteria are probably too strict.[5] We have found that in the absence of gross infiltrates and obviously infected secretions, many donor lungs can be used which would otherwise not meet established criteria and which would therefore be considered marginal.[5] Nevertheless, the loosening of donor criteria is unlikely to significantly increase the number of donor lungs that are presently needed for transplantation in North America.

The problem of donor lung shortage is far more acute in the pediatric population. The reasons for this are many, including the facts that size is much more of an issue in the pediatric lung transplant patient and the lungs are often injured in many potential pediatric donors. Though several successful series of pediatric lung transplantation have been reported,[6–11] the extent of use of lung transplantation in the pediatric population is limited by the lack of adequate donors. A possible solution for the pediatric lung transplant candidate is the use of a lobe or segment from an adult living related or cadaveric donor; the so called reduced-size or reduced-volume lung transplant. Not only does this technique allow for living related transplantation with its associated immunologic advantages, but multiple lobes from a single cadaveric donor could potentially be used for several recipients.

There is a great deal of precedent in other organ systems for utilizing a living relative as a source of intraoperative support or of organs for transplantation. The initial use of a parent as an oxygenator for a child was in

congenital cardiac operations done by Lillehei and his colleagues at the University of Minnesota.[12] These innovative physicians were able to utilize a parent to provide adequate oxygenation of the child's blood during operative repair of certain cardiac defects. There was some controversy, however, because of the potential 200% mortality for these procedures. This technique was no longer necessary once the pump oxygenator was developed.

Living related kidney donation was the first area where relatives were used as a source of organs. It still remains a very successful means of kidney transplantation with a mortality of virtually 0% for the donor and is a widely accepted practice. More recently, living related liver transplantation for children with end-stage liver disease was developed by Dr. Christoph Broelsch and his colleagues.[13] As of May 11, 1992 surgeons at the University of Chicago Medical Center had performed 42 living related reduced-size liver transplants. Of the 42 transplant recipients 37 survived and none of the donors died during harvesting.

We became interested in the concept of using living related lung tissue as a means of expanding the pediatric donor lung pool and to provide elective transplantation for children with end-stage lung disease. It was our feeling that indications would at least initially be restricted to individuals who required only single lung transplantation believing that getting two segments of lung for both sides would be very difficult. However, even this formidable undertaking was recently accomplished when Dr. Vaughn Starnes performed a bilateral reduced-size lung transplant using lobes from both parents in a young patient with cystic fibrosis (personal communication).

Among the major issues to be overcome are the proper indications for reduced-size transplantation. For instance, it may be that patients with pulmonary hypertension will have a difficult time undergoing single lung reduced-size transplantation. There has been a great deal of controversy in the adult literature about whether single lung transplants can be used in individuals with pulmonary hypertension. Though there have been successful reports[3] of single lung transplantation for pulmonary hypertension, many centers report difficulty using single lungs in these patients since the transplanted organ often floods. Another major clinical issue which needs to be addressed is just how much growth there will be in a mature lobe placed as a single lung into a growing child. Though this monograph will review laboratory investigation in this area, there is not enough clinical experience to know how much, if any, growth to expect in a reduced-size lung transplant.

Finally, there is the unanswered question of whether the mature lobar transplant is better or worse than a cadaveric immature whole lung transplant for the pediatric or neonatal recipient. Though there has been some laboratory investigation in this area the clinical experience with lung transplantation in children is not extensive enough to yield good long-term data about growth and function of cadaveric immature whole lung transplants.

We believe that the potential for this innovative approach to pediatric lung transplantation is vast. It is unclear that there will ever be enough pediatric cadaveric lung donors to provide enough organs for most infants and children requiring lung transplantation. Reduced-size lung transplantation is a way to immediately expand the donor lung pool not only for children but also for small adults with limited thoracic cavities. Although there has been a modest amount of laboratory investigation in this area, clinical experience is limited. The purpose of this monograph is: 1) to discuss issues unique to pediatric lung transplantation, 2) to review the laboratory background for reduced-size lung transplantation, 3) to describe the small amount of clinical work that has been done so far, and 4) to discuss the ethics of living related lung transplantation.

REFERENCES

1. Cooper JD, Grossman RF, Halloran P, Patterson GA, Todd TRJ. Unilateral lung transplantation for pulmonary fibrosis. N Engl J Med 1986; 314:1140-4.

2. Morgan WG, Lima O, Goldberg M, Ayabe H, Groman A, Cooper JD. Improved bronchial healing in canine left lung reimplantation using omental pedicle wrap. J Thorac Cardiovasc Surg 1983; 85:134-49.

3. Spray TL, Mallory GB, Canter CE, Huddleston CB, Kaiser LR. Pediatric lung transplantation for pulmonary hypertension and congenital heart disease. Ann Thorac Surg 1992; 54:216-25.

4. Egan TM, Kaiser LR, Cooper JD. "Lung Transplantation" in Current Problems in Surgery. Wells SA (Ed.) (Chicago: Year Book Medical Publishers), 1989.

5. Kron IL, Tribble CG, Kern JA et al. Successful transplantation of marginally acceptable thoracic organs. Ann Surg 1993; In Press.

6. Michler RE, Rose EA. Pediatric heart and heart-lung transplantation. Ann Thorac Surg 1991; 52:708-9.

7. Smyth RL, Scott JP, Whitehead B et al. The use of heart-lung transplantation in management of terminal respiratory complications of cystic fibrosis. Transplant Proc 1990; 22:1472-3.

8. Smyth RL, Scott JP, Whitehead B et al. Heart-lung transplantation in children. Transplant Proc 1990; 22:1470-1.

9. Starnes VA, Marshall SE, Lewiston NJ et al. Heart-lung transplantation in infants, children, and adolescents. J Pediatr Surg 1991; 26:434-8.

10. Armitage JM, Kormos RL, Flicker FJ. Pediatric pulmonary transplantation: the University of Pittsburgh experience. J Heart-Lung Transplant 1991; 10:162.

11. M'etras D, Shennib H, Kreitmann B, Camboulives J et al. Double-lung transplantation in children: a report of 20 cases. Ann Thorac Surg 1993; 55:352-7.

12. Warden HE, Cohen ME, Lillehei CW. Controlled cross-circulation for intracardiac surgery. J Thorac Surg 1954; 28:331-43.

13. Broelsch CE, Whitington PF, Emond JL et al. Liver transplantation in children from living related donors, surgical techniques and results. Ann Surg 1991; 214(4):428-37.

PEDIATRIC LUNG TRANSPLANTATION: OVERVIEW, INDICATIONS, PHYSIOLOGY

Charles B. Huddleston
Thomas L. Spray

INTRODUCTION

Barely a decade has passed since the first successful lung transplant by the group at Toronto in November of 1983.[1] Over that period of time the number of transplant centers performing this procedure has burgeoned significantly with greater than 1500 patients receiving either double or single lung transplants over the past five years.[2] Improvement in the results obtained in adults and refinement in techniques have led to the application of this treatment to the pediatric population, although they account for less than 10% of all lung transplants performed. Children differ from adults in a number of fundamental ways, and these differences are magnified as the age of the transplant recipient drops to less than one year. This chapter will deal with all issues of pulmonary transplantation in children and how they differ from those of adults.

Reduced-size Lung Transplantation, edited by John A. Kern, M.D. and Irving L. Kron, M.D.; © 1993 R.G. Landes Company.

INDICATIONS

As in adults the indications for lung transplantation in pediatric patients include end-stage lung disease of the restrictive or obstructive type or end-stage pulmonary vascular disease, either primary or secondary. Secondary pulmonary vascular disease associated with correctable congenital cardiac defects may be an indication for lung transplantation if cardiac repair can be undertaken at the time of pulmonary transplantation. Severe functional limitation and an anticipated life expectancy of 12 to 18 months without transplantation are additional requirements for consideration of transplantation.

The types of pulmonary disease seen in children which would require transplantation early in life are significantly different from those observed in adults. Emphysema, a common indication for pulmonary transplantation in adults is a very infrequent cause of end-stage lung disease in the pediatric population. Similarly, pulmonary fibrosis is a rare isolated entity in children and it is unusual for fibrotic pulmonary disease in pediatric patients to progress sufficiently to require transplantation in the first 16 to 18 years of life. Thus, the disease entities enjoying the best results following transplantation in the adult population are eliminated from consideration in the pediatric age group. Although unusual types of pulmonary fibrosis do occur in pediatric patients which might require lung transplantation the slowly progressive nature of these diseases often results in survival past the pediatric age range. A summary of some indications for pediatric lung transplantation is given in Table 1.

Primary pulmonary vascular disease with pulmonary hypertension is usually not severe enough to cause deterioration and death in patients under the age of 16 years. Therefore, a relatively small proportion of these patients

---

Table 1. Pediatric Indications for Lung Transplantation

Pulmonary Fibrosis
    Usual interstitial fibrosis (UIP)
    Desquamative interstitial fibrosis (DIP)
    Pulmonary alveolar proteinosis
    Idiopathic pulmonary alveolar microlithiasis
    Cystic fibrosis
    Radiation-induced pulmonary fibrosis
    Obliterative bronchiolitis
    Bronchopulmonary dysplasia
    Congenital surfactant protein deficiencies
    Auto-immune diseases
    ? Acute respiratory distress syndrome ?

Pulmonary Vascular Disease
    Primary pulmonary hypertension
    Pulmonary hypertension after corrected congenital heart disease
    Pulmonary hypertension and correctable congenital heart disease (Eisenmenger's syndrome)
    "Inadequate" pulmonary vascular bed
    Pulmonary atresia, ventricular septal defect, no central pulmonary arteries
    Congenital diaphragmatic hernia

present with progressive dilatation and syncope in childhood such that they may be considered for pulmonary transplantation. However, because of the unpredictable course and high incidence of sudden death in those patients with severe elevations of pulmonary artery pressure and vascular resistance we have undertaken a policy of listing them for transplantation at presentation even in the absence of symptoms. A more common subgroup of patients includes those with secondary pulmonary vascular disease coexisting with significant corrected or uncorrected congenital heart disease. The association of pulmonary hypertension and congenital heart disease may result in progressive right ventricular dysfunction and cyanosis, and if palliative surgical procedures are exhausted and progressive disability is noted, pulmonary transplantation and repair of the congenital cardiac defects may be indicated.[3] However, timing for transplantation is very difficult in that these children often live for a very long period of time beyond the time that cyanosis might appear.

A unique pediatric population that may require pulmonary transplantation are children with cystic fibrosis. The majority of cystic fibrosis patients survive into adulthood with adequate medical management. Nevertheless, a small proportion of children may require transplantation before age 16 to 18 years. Relative indications for consideration of lung transplantation in the cystic fibrosis group include an increasing frequency of hospitalizations for antibiotic therapy, progressive weight loss in older patients or a persistent lack of weight gain in younger patients despite adequate nutritional supplementation, an increase in oxygen dependence or rising pCO_2 with worsening exercise tolerance, and an FEV_1 of less than 30% of predicted. Children with cystic fibrosis meeting indications for transplantation are, in most cases, quite debilitated. Multiple antibiotic-resistant organisms may be present in the tracheobronchial tree complicating transplantation and increasing the risk of posttransplantation sepsis.[4]

An interesting and challenging group of patients potentially treatable with lung transplantation are neonates with congenital diaphragmatic hernia. The prognosis for these infants as a whole is poor with a mortality of 50%, and those diagnosed in utero by ultrasonography may have a mortality of greater than 75%. Although extracorporeal membrane oxygenation (ECMO) support prior to or following repair has improved the survival rates, 20–50% of these patients will not be able to be weaned from ECMO and subsequently die.[5] Most of these deaths are due to pulmonary hypertension and pulmonary hypoplasia. Theoretically, a single lung transplant on the affected side could provide a sufficient addition of pulmonary vascular bed to reduce pulmonary hypertension and also additional pulmonary parenchyma to get the neonate over the critical early stage of life. Once the lung on the unaffected side has had time to grow and develop, the transplanted lung would presumably no longer be necessary and could potentially be removed at a time when growth would allow for compensated expansion of the native lung. Further, this is the setting in which lobar transplantation from a larger donor or even living related lung donation is feasible.[6]

A particularly difficult group of children occasionally considered for lung transplantation are those who develop acute severe respiratory distress syndrome from a variety of causes such as viral or necrotizing pneumonia and idiopathic drug reactions. In general, these children are otherwise normal and up until their acute illness have been in good health. ECMO has been increasingly utilized in pediatric patients over the past several years when the lung disease has progressed to the point of requiring very unfavorable ventilator settings to provide nominally acceptable gas exchange. Since 1986 over 400 pediatric patients have been placed on ECMO for this reason with survival (weaning from ECMO) rates of 30–50%. One could infer from these data that at least half of these patients would be potential candidates for lung transplantation if donor lungs were available.

However, the increasingly long waiting times for donor lungs and lack of an acute status classification with United Network of Organ Sharing (UNOS) for lung transplant candidates makes the likelihood of receiving organs in a timely fashion poor. Our own experience with one child and experience at other centers suggest that single lung transplantation will not succeed in patients with acute lung disease because of ventilation/perfusion mismatch with a well perfused and ventilated transplanted lung compromised by persistent perfusion of the native, poorly ventilated lung. The options, therefore, would be bilateral lung transplantation, single lung transplantation with banding of the branch pulmonary artery to the native lung or single lung transplantation with pneumonectomy of the contralateral lung.

Relative contraindications to lung transplantation in the pediatric population include severe scoliosis that significantly affects chest wall mechanics, poorly controlled diabetes mellitus or left heart dysfunction. Prior thoracotomy, particularly if accompanied by a surgical pleurectomy, complicates the transplant procedure because of dense adhesions and bleeding. We have found the use of aprotonin to be extremely useful in this circumstance and would not necessarily exclude these patients from consideration for transplantation. Others have used epsilon-aminocaproic acid or tranexamic acid with good results as well. Steroid dependence in high doses may be associated with increased risk of poor bronchial healing and sepsis following transplantation and is, thus, a relative contraindication to lung transplantation. Nevertheless, small to moderate doses of steroids are not associated with significant healing complications and the consideration of patients must be individualized.

As in all transplant procedures the family support of the pediatric patient is of primary importance. The family must be committed to long-term health care and be willing to comply with multiple medical interventions in order to ensure the success of the transplant and the long-term outcome.

Because of the smaller size of children it was hoped that waiting times for lungs for pediatric patients would be significantly shorter than that for adults. In spite of this theoretical advantage, however, it has become clear that the average waiting time for pediatric donor lungs is now at least six months to one year and significant mortality occurs in children awaiting transplantation. In one patient in our series who was two weeks old at the time of listing for lung transplantation, ECMO was required for pulmonary support and the patient was maintained on this for one month before neurologic complications precluded transplantation. While this child was listed, no donor organs became available despite no other patients of similar size range being listed in the United States. Thus, there is an apparent significant shortage of potential donors for the newborn age population despite the availability of infant heart donors for similar size patients. Many adult patients are small due to their chronic illness and small lungs can be utilized in significantly larger adults due to the capacity of the lung to expand to the pleural cavity. Adult transplant recipients take up lungs from pediatric-age donors that could potentially be utilized in a pediatric-age recipient. In addition, there are relatively fewer pediatric donors available and large lungs from adult patients may not be suitable for use in pediatric recipients. These issues have established the need for early listing for potential recipients and the need for a transplant center to develop the capacity to treat these end-stage patients for prolonged periods of time.

TECHNIQUE OF LUNG TRANSPLANTATION

The technical aspects of pulmonary transplantation in children are similar to those in adult patients. Several modifications of the adult technique are necessary, however, to account for the size variation in children. The very thin and tenuous nature of omentum in many malnourished and small pediatric patients has led to abandonment of its use for bronchial wrapping in pediatric patients. In addition, many children have had a previous gastrostomy for feeding purposes and entering the abdomen and taking down adhesions for mobilization of the omentum is complicated. We have utilized pericardial pedicles taken down at the time of opening the pericardium to place patients on cardiopulmonary bypass as a means of wrapping the bronchial anastomoses in our patients. Although it is clear from adult data that a bronchial wrap is not required for good tracheobronchial healing,[7] wrapping the bronchus with pericardial pedicles may prevent disruption of an adjacent pulmonary arterial anastomosis if anastomotic bronchial disruption occurs. A recent improvement in the rate of anastomotic bronchial complications even without a bronchial wrap suggests that wrapping of the bronchus is not necessary and, therefore, if pericardium is not readily available no bronchial wrap is utilized.[8]

The bronchial anastomoses have been performed in an end-to-end fashion in children utilizing absorbable suture material in hopes of preventing residual foreign body in the airway and maximizing growth potential. We have not utilized telescoping bronchial anastomoses unless donor and recipient size discrepancy is severe. As might be expected in children, a significant incidence of bronchial anastomotic complications has occurred with either disruption or stenosis of bronchial suture lines and bronchomalacia. Localized airway complications are managed with placement of silastic stents (Hood Labs, Pembroke, MA) which have been successful in preventing progressive stenosis of anastomoses in our pediatric patients. In the limited experience with pediatric lung transplantation to date, it is unclear that the technique of bronchial anastomosis or the age of the patient significantly alters the incidence or severity of bronchial complications.[9]

The majority of children who undergo pediatric lung transplantation require the use of cardiopulmonary bypass for the procedure. The use of cardiopulmonary bypass eliminates the need for double lumen endotracheal tubes or bronchial blockers which are cumbersome and often not suitable or available for use in very small children or young adults. The copious secretions in cystic fibrosis patients make single lung ventilation difficult and may result in contamination of the newly transplanted lung. In addition, the hyperinflation of the lungs along with the relatively small size has made it difficult to dissect the hilum in many patients at the time of transplantation. We use a bilateral transverse thoracotomy incision and routinely place patients on cardiopulmonary bypass for both bilateral or single lung transplantation (Fig. 1). The use of the bilateral transverse thoracotomy incision has provided excellent exposure for take down of pleural adhesions and for access to the heart and mediastinum for repair of congenital cardiac defects.[10] In addition, it is possible to remove both lungs and to irrigate and clean the blind trachea with antibiotic solution before implantation of the donor lungs thus diminishing the contamination of the transplanted lungs in cystic fibrosis patients. Because the femoral artery and vein are often small in children we have utilized direct aortic and right atrial cannulation through the bilateral transverse thoracotomy in almost all instances for lung transplantation with or without cardiac repair. Although significant periods of cardiopulmonary bypass have been necessary in many children, there have not been any complications of cardiopulmonary bypass noted in these children to date.

TRANSPLANTATION IN INFANTS

Just as the success of transplantation of lungs in adults led to attempts in older children, the success in this area prompted consideration of transplantation in young children, infants and even neonates. The issues that have come up in this group of patients include growth potential of the graft, the use of reduced size adult organs, and the feasibility of living related donors.

GROWTH

Growth of the lung from birth to adulthood occurs as a result of an increase in number of alveoli and an increase in the size of the alveoli. Alveoli multiply in number rapidly for 2–3 years, with growth diminishing in an exponential fashion after that, essentially stopping altogether at about the age of 8 years. The number of alveoli increases about ten-fold over this period of time. Alveolar diameter, on the other hand, remains relatively constant up to 8 years increasing from 210 μm to 230 μm. Beyond that it increases in size to 280 μm by the age of 25. Between the ages 8 to 25 the lung volume doubles; this increase is accounted for by the increase in size of the alveolus itself.[11–13]

There is fairly good experimental data demonstrating that the transplantation of immature lungs in immature recipients will result in normal growth with an increase in alveolar number in these transplanted immature lungs accompanying a period of somatic growth of the animal.[14–16] Furthermore, the lobar bronchi and the pulmonary arteries grow to a size appropriate for the size of the animal. Denervation of the lung does not influence this growth. However, when mature or adult lungs are used for transplantation in growing animals there is some lung growth but not by an increase in the number or size of alveoli. This growth appears to be on the basis of an increase in cellular and connective tissue elements[17] which obviously will not contribute to the ventilatory capacity of that lung.

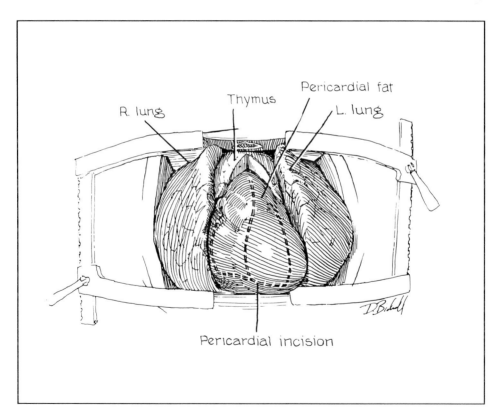

Fig. 1. Transverse bilateral thoracotomy incision with exposure of the lungs and heart for cannulation. Dotted lines show the pericardial incisions for take-down of bilateral pericardial pedicles to wrap the bronchial anastomoses.

PHYSIOLOGY

Pulmonary vascular resistance

The effect of denervation on pulmonary vascular resistance (PVR) is to cause it to rise when blood flow to the denervated lung is increased. This is reversible and as this response to denervation diminishes the PVR will fall. There is experimental evidence to suggest that mature lobar transplants would better accept the majority of the cardiac output than immature whole lung transplant in terms of the response of the pulmonary vascular bed. The differences between immature and mature lung transplants in this area may be related to the degree of pulmonary maturation at the time of denervation or transplantation. The "immature" lungs involved in these studies are in very young animals. Presumably a donor lung from an 8–10 year old would be less likely to show these characteristics.[18,19]

Airway compliance

In general, mature or normal adult lungs have a higher compliance than immature or very young lungs. Following transplantation the compliance falls somewhat. Airway resistance rises in both the mature transplanted lobe and the native immature whole lung following transplantation. The transplanted mature lobe will be preferentially ventilated relative to the native lung because of this reduced compliance. This is manifested by lower pCO_2 in the pulmonary vein of the transplanted lung compared to that of the native lung.[6] As a normal lung grows and matures, there is an "alveolization" of the terminal bronchioli such that they become respiratory bronchioli. The terminal bronchioli thus become a relatively more proximal structure in the bronchial tree as the number of respiratory alveoli per unit lung tissue increases. This is presumably the explanation for increased compliance in the mature lung.[20]

Thus, it would seem from experimental data that in the setting of using a single lung for transplant in a small infant or neonate, a lobar transplant from a mature donor would theoretically be a better option in the short term from the standpoint of both pulmonary vascular and airway compliance. However, the potential for growth is limited and how this might impact on the long-term functional capacity of the transplant recipient is unknown.

ANATOMY FOR REDUCED-SIZE LUNG TRANSPLANT

Animal studies

Experimental animal studies have varied depending upon the species and relative sizes of donor and recipient animals in terms of which lobe or segment of lung has proven to be most useful.[6,16–19,21,22] Table 2 lists some of these. Pigs would appear to tolerate lung transplantation reasonably well and a model using the left lower lobe as the left lung has been successful for producing survivors of 12 or more weeks.[19]

Table 2. Animal Models of Reduced-size Lung Transplants

Animal	Center	Donor Portion	Recipient Portion	Size Diff. (body wt.)
Pigs	UCSF	Apical Segment LUL	Left Lung	25%
Pigs	Univ Va	LLL	Left Lung	20%
Pigs	UCSF	LLL	Left Lung	30%
Sheep	Harvard	RUL, LUL	Left Lung	6%
Beagles	Northwestern	LLL	Left Lung	33%

Human transplantation

Dissections carried out by Jennings et al[23] indicate that for use in a neonate, the adult right middle lobe or anterior segment of the right middle lobe have the most favorable hilar anatomy and size match for the left lung when rotated 180°. For transplantation into older children where the size discrepancy is not quite as large the adult upper lobes would provide quite favorable hilar anatomy. To date, seven children have undergone reduced-size lung transplants (personal communication, V. Starnes) and one child has had lobar transplants bilaterally, one from each parent.[24] Six of these have been right lung transplants (four right upper lobe, one right middle lobe, one right lower lobe donors) and one was a left lung transplant using the left upper lobe of the donor. Four of these seven children received their organ from a living related donor, a parent in all cases. All seven transplants were "technical" successes. Three of these patients died in the early postoperative period and two others have died later in the first postoperative year. Although these results are not spectacular by any measure, all seven patients were very high risk. Two patients were on ECMO support prior to transplantation and two were ventilated.[25]

Congenital diaphragmatic hernia remains a very lethal condition due to pulmonary hypoplasia and pulmonary hypertension. Mortality rates for this condition range from 20 to 60% in various centers. Those requiring ECMO for support in the perioperative period are at even greater risk. These neonates represent a group that might benefit from reduced-size lung transplant or even living related donor lung transplant. It is conceivable that once out of the neonatal period and after the contralateral lung has had time to grow, the transplanted lung could be removed when compensatory growth of the native lung could ultimately result in nearly normal ventilatory capacity.[26] All immunosuppressive drugs could then be discontinued. However, as other treatment modalities for congenital diaphragmatic hernia are developed (such as nitric oxide and exogenous surfactant), the mortality for these neonates may drop, reducing the need for lung transplantation.

IMMUNOSUPPRESSION

Our immunosuppression protocol for pediatric lung transplantation has evolved over the course of the program development at St. Louis Children's Hospital. Initially, protocols used for lung transplantation were quite similar to those used for infant and pediatric heart transplantation in our institution. Azathioprine is begun at 2 mg/kg intravenously before the transplant procedure and cyclosporine is begun at 0.25 to 0.5 mg/kg intravenously over the first three hours after transplant and then the dosage is decreased to 1.5 to 2.5 mg/hr to maintain whole blood immunofluorescence cyclosporine levels at 300 to 500 ng/ml in the immediate postoperative period. Early in our experience, methylprednisolone at 1 mg/kg/d intravenously and azathioprine at 3 mg/kg/d orally or intravenously were begun immediately following the transplant. Because of an evident increase in septic complications with higher-dose steroids the protocol has been altered and we now use antithymocyte globulin (ATG, Atgam®) at a dose of 10 mg/kg/d for the first 5–7 days following the transplant, with an associated decrease in maintenance steroid administration to 0.5 mg/kg/d. In addition, antiviral agents are administered for documented cytomegalovirus (CMV) infection based on buffy coat cultures from blood and tracheobronchial washings or for situations in which there is a CMV mismatch between donor and recipient. Ganciclovir® may be used prophylactically for the first six weeks following transplantation in the hope of delaying significant viral infection, especially with Epstein-Barr virus, until major rejection episodes have subsided.

Rejection episodes are diagnosed by increasing infiltrates on chest radiography, fever, leukocytosis, a decrease in peripheral arterial oxygen saturation and ventilatory function, or by the development of new pleural effusions. Transbronchial lung biopsy is done to confirm the diagnosis and to evaluate the effectiveness of treatment. Rejection episodes are treated with bolus steroids. Rejection refractory to steroids is treated with another seven day course of ATG at a dose of 10 mg/kg/d.

Other immunosuppressive protocols have been described for pediatric lung transplantation.[27,28] The protocols use either FK506 or are based on standard triple therapy with azathioprine, cyclosporine, and prednisone. From the limited number of pediatric transplants performed to date it is unclear whether there is a significant superiority of one immunosuppression protocol over another; however, the availability of newer immunosuppressive agents such as FK506 may make dosage and administration easier in children, who may require multiple divided doses of cyclosporine to maintain adequate cyclosporine levels and for patients with cystic fibrosis who may have difficulty with gastrointestinal absorption of cyclosporine.

REJECTION SURVEILLANCE

Bronchoscopy is performed frequently in the early postoperative period after lung transplantation to assess bronchial healing. Despite some technical difficulty in obtaining transbronchial biopsies in small infants, it is possible to perform blind transbronchial biopsy through a rigid bronchoscope in infants using a modified cardiac bioptome or directed biopsies using the same technique with fluoroscopic control with sampling of at least two areas of the transplanted lungs. Three to six specimens are taken at each biopsy. In order to assess the magnitude of rejection and the evidence of resolution of rejection episodes frequent biopsies are performed if there is any change in the clinical status of the patient. A routine surveillance biopsy is obtained approximately one week after the transplant and then one to three additional biopsies are performed in the first three months following transplantation and every six months thereafter.

If inadequate tissue is obtained on transbronchial biopsy in the setting of clinically suspected rejection an open lung biopsy is performed. In addition, progressively decreasing respiratory function by spirometry without evidence for rejection on transbronchial biopsy has been considered an indication for open lung biopsy to determine the presence of bronchiolitis obliterans.

Pulmonary function tests are performed two weeks after transplant and then weekly. Exercise stress tests are performed at six weeks, three months, and six months following the transplantation. To aid in the identification of early rejection episodes patients and their families are taught the techniques of home spirometry and oximetry and report any change in daily values. In addition, daily rehabilitation therapy for the first three months following transplantation is considered a critical component of the post-transplant medical care.

RESULTS FROM ST. LOUIS CHILDREN'S HOSPITAL

The experience of the pediatric lung transplant program at St. Louis Children's Hospital, Washington University, from August 1990 to March 1993 includes 30 patients who have undergone 33 transplant procedures (Table 3). There have been 8 single lung transplants and 22 bilateral sequential transplants in this series. One of the patients receiving a single lung transplant actually had the right lower lobe of a cadaveric donor used as a right lung transplant (Fig. 2). This donor had provided a heart and single lung transplant for another recipient in our program. Three patients have required retransplantation, two with bilateral sequential technique and one with an en bloc technique. The primary diagnoses of the 30 patients who underwent transplantation in this series are summarized in Table 3. The age of recipients has been from 1.5 to 23 years with a mean of 11.41 ± 2.39 years. All three retransplant patients have died confirming the very high mortality for retransplant pulmonary operations noted by

Miller and Patterson.[29] Seven patients died during the posttransplant hospitalization and three additional patients died late after transplantation: one from a lymphoproliferative disorder 10 weeks following bilateral sequential transplantation and two with bronchiolitis obliterans, one of whom died before a retransplant donor was available and the other following retransplantation for progressive bronchiolitis obliterans. Characteristics

Table 3. Pediatric Lung Transplants at St. Louis Children's Hospital August 1990–March 1993

Diagnosis	Number	Survivors (%)
Cystic Fibrosis	11	7 (64%)
Pulmonary Fibrosis	6	6 100%)
Pulmonary Hypertension		
Primary	5	3 (60%)
Congenital Heart Disease	5	2 (40%)
Respiratory Distress Syndrome	1	0 (0%)
Re-transplant	3	0 (0%)
Total (30 patients)	33	18 (60%)

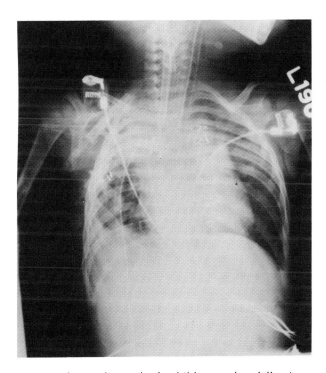

Fig. 2. Chest radiograph of a child seven days following transplantation of a cadaveric right lower lobe in the right chest as a single lung transplant.

Table 4. Pediatric Lung Transplant Patients

Diagnosis	PT	Age (yrs)	Type	Pre-op Support	Outcome
Cystic Fibrosis					
	BT	12	Bilateral	None	Late death six months, OB
	AS	18	Bilateral	None	Retranspl. early, died (sepsis)
	JP	17	Bilateral	None	Died early (LPD, sepsis)
	GW	13	Bilateral	None	Retranspl. early, died (sepsis)
	BC	12	Bilateral	None	Alive
	SA	9	Bilateral	None	Alive
	ML	16	Bilateral	None	Alive
	AM	9	Bilateral	None	Alive
	DB	15	Bilateral	None	Alive
	JN	10	Bilateral	Ventilated	Alive
	SS	16	Bilateral	Ventilated	Alive
1° Pulmonary Htn					
	BB	15	Single R	None	Alive
	AS	1.7	Bilateral	ECMO	Alive
	AL	1.5	Bilateral	ECMO	Died eight weeks posttx (LPD)
	RM	1.6	Bilateral	None	Died six weeks posttx (graft failure)
	WK	15	Single L	None	Alive
Eisenmenger's					
	JD	23	Single R	None	Alive
	BD	11	Single R	None	Retranspl. 10 mo. later; died (sepsis)
Heart Disease					
	TK	5	Bilateral	None	Alive
	GC	10	Bilateral	None	Died in OR due to bleeding
	JS	12	Bilateral	None	Died six weeks posttx (ruptured pseudoaneurysm of RVOT)
	AL	5	Single L	None	Alive
	MW	2	Lobar RLL	ECMO	Died one weeks postop (graft failure)
Pulmonary Fibrosis					
	DF	11	Bilateral	None	Alive
	JM	17	Single L	Ventilated	Alive
	LB	5	Bilateral	Ventilated	Alive
	JD	6	Bilateral	None	Alive
	DS	13	Bilateral	None	Alive
	BB	8	Bilateral	None	Alive
ARDS					
	KE	13	Single L	ECMO	Died one week posttx (MOF)

of the transplanted patients are listed in Table 4.

The best results in our series have been in patients with pulmonary fibrosis. All of these patients have survived. The underlying etiology of pulmonary fibrosis in these children has been quite diverse—bronchopulmonary dysplasia, interstitial pneumonitis, histiocytosis-X, bronchiolitis obliterans and two with pulmonary fibrosis following bone marrow transplantation for acute myelogenous leukemia. Seven of the 12 patients who underwent lung transplant for pulmonary hypertension with or without significant cardiac disease survived. Two of these had VSD closure and single lung transplantation for Eisenmenger's syndrome, three underwent bilateral lung transplantation/VSD closure/pulmonary homograft reconstruction of the right ventricular outflow tract to the transplanted lungs, two underwent ligation of a patent ductus arteriosus and single or double lung transplant, one underwent single lung transplant with heart transplant and four underwent atrial septal defect closure and lung transplant. Of the 11 patients with cystic fibrosis transplanted 7 have survived. One patient transplanted for acute respiratory distress syndrome died early posttransplant.

There have been seven early deaths following pediatric lung transplantation. The causes have been sepsis (2), intraoperative hemorrhage (1), ARDS (2), lymphoproliferative disease (2). Three have died late after transplant: two due to bronchiolitis obliterans and one from rupture of a pseudoaneurysm of the right ventricle. Thus, the early survival has been 74% and the one-year survival has been 64%.

Apart from those mentioned above, complications seen early after transplantation include hemorrhage (2), phrenic nerve injury (2) and bronchial anastomotic problems (6). Of the 47 bronchial anastomoses at risk, complications developed in seven: strictures (3), complete disruption (1), partial disruption (1), bronchomalacia (2). Five stents have been placed for treatment of these complications including one patient who required bilateral bronchial stents (Fig. 3). Active Aspergillus infection was noted in the bronchus that completely disrupted and transplant pneumonectomy was required. The patient with partial disruption of her bronchial anastomosis was treated with antibiotics only and the disruption healed very slowly over time.

The major late complication occurring after discharge has been bronchiolitis obliterans. We have used spirometry data as screening information for this diagnosis. When there is a sustained consistent drop in the FEV_1, the patients are evaluated with computed tomography of the chest and bronchoscopy with transbronchial biopsy. If the histology from this does not produce a satisfactory diagnosis open lung biopsy is performed. Seven of the 22 patients surviving the early posttransplant period have developed bronchiolitis obliterans and two of these have died. The other five patients have had their disease arrested with a 10 day course of ATG and an increase in their steroid and cyclosporine doses. Although the etiology of bronchiolitis obliterans is unclear we have taken the view that it is a manifestation of chronic rejection. When diagnosed "early" we have had reasonable success in stopping its progression. The two patients who died had a fall in FEV_1 to an average of 15% of predicted whereas those surviving under treatment had an average FEV_1 of 50% of predicted at the time of diagnosis. Presumably this represents the effects of treatment earlier in the course of the disease. For children too small to cooperate for pulmonary function testing we have no reliable screening tests for this complication.

DISCUSSION

Although combined heart and lung transplantation has been performed in several centers in pediatric recipients there have been relatively few reported series of pediatric pulmonary transplantation.[10,25,28,30–35] The largest group of pediatric pulmonary transplant recipients for cystic fibrosis has been reported by M'etras and associates from the Montreal/Marseille lung transplant program.[30] Overall

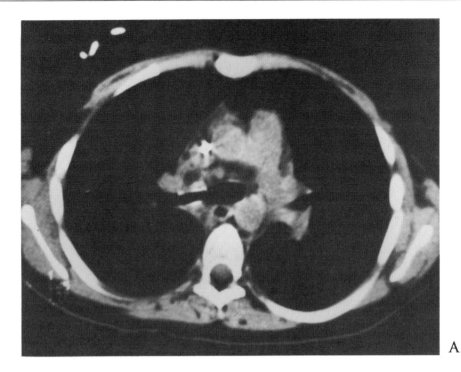

A

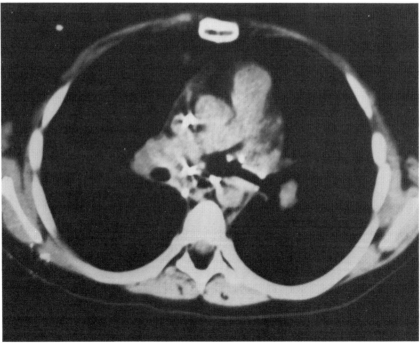

B

Fig. 3A. A view of the chest CT scan showing the stent placement in the right mainstem bronchus placed 10 weeks following bilateral lung transplantation for cystic fibrosis in a 12-year-old girl. She developed stenosis at the suture line in her bronchial anastomosis. B. View of the chest CT scan on the same patient taken on the same day. She had developed partial disruption of the bronchial anastomosis which led to stenosis of the left mainstem bronchus. The stent can be easily seen in this view.

results with lung transplantation in this group of children have been excellent with 80% early and late survival rates up to two years following the transplant procedure. These authors have not noted a significantly increased incidence of rejection or infection in the pediatric transplant recipients as compared to adult transplant patients.

A small number of pediatric pulmonary recipients have been reported from the group in Pittsburgh and early results with the use of FK506 and azathioprine and low-dose steroids have been excellent with approximately 80% hospital survival and no late deaths reported.[35] Follow-up ranges from six months to six years although the majority of pediatric pulmonary

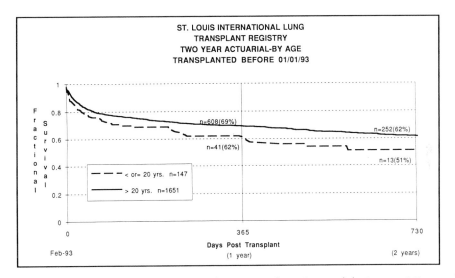

Fig. 4. Actuarial survival following lung transplantation—adult (age > 20) vs. pediatric (age < 20). In general, the results in adults have been slightly better than in children. The number of pediatric patients at two years posttransplant is small making this time in follow-up difficult to interpret.

Table 5. St. Louis International Lung Transplant Registry Pediatric Transplants (0–20 years)

Group	Age in Years				
	0 - 5	6 - 10	11-16	17-20	Total
Single	4	6	16	13	39
Bilateral	8	14	31	41	94
En-bloc Double	1	3	9	8	21
Unknown			2	2	4
Total	13	23	58	64	158

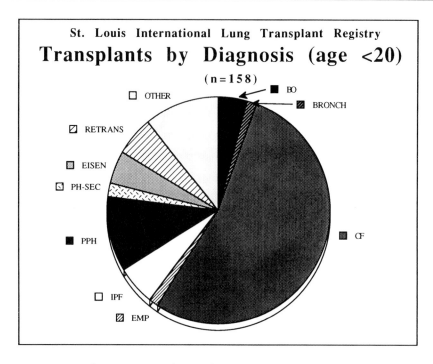

Fig. 5. Transplantation according to diagnosis in pediatric patients. CF=cystic fibrosis, PPH=primary pulmonary hypertension, PH-SEC=pulmonary hypertension of a secondary nature, IPF= idiopathic pulmonary fibrosis, BRONCH=bronchiectasis, EMP=emphysema, EISEN=Eisenmenger's syndrome, RE-TRANS=retransplant, B.O.=bronchiolitis obliterans.

transplants have had less than two years of follow-up. As noted in the St. Louis Children's Hospital series, complications have included phrenic palsy, bronchial stenosis, post-transplant lymphoproliferative disease and frequent viral infections.

Review of the pediatric transplants reported to the St. Louis International Lung Transplant Registry confirm that the results reported with pediatric lung transplantation are not yet comparable to the results noted in adults (Fig. 4). Of the 1798 transplants reported to the Lung Transplant Registry by January 1, 1993, 158 (8.8%) were in patients less than 21 years of age.[2] Of those 158, 122 (77%) were in children 11–20 years of age. Ninety-four of the 158 were bilateral sequential transplants, 21 were en bloc doubles, 39 were singles and 4 unknown (Table 5). Figures

5 and 6 compare the transplants by diagnosis in the adult and pediatric groups with the division coming arbitrarily at age 20. The majority of transplants in adults are being performed for emphysema, a disease not seen commonly in children. This group stands out as that which has the best result thus far of any of the diagnostic groups receiving transplantation with actuarial survival rates of 74% at one year and 68% at two years. Cystic fibrosis, on the other hand, is becoming an increasingly frequent diagnosis for lung transplantation and is the largest single indication for transplantation in the pediatric group. The overall actuarial survival of pediatric cystic fibrosis transplant recipients reported to the Registry shows a one-year survival of approximately 70% and a two-year survival of 40%. Only a few transplanted children,

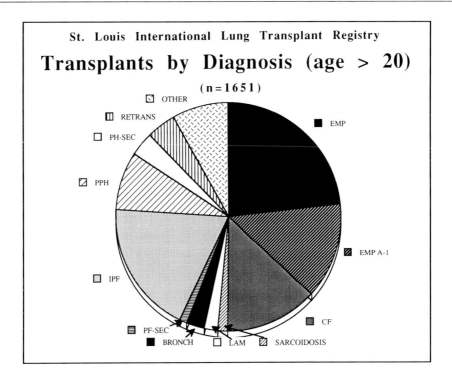

Fig. 6. Transplantation according to diagnosis in adult patients. CF=cystic fibrosis, PPH=primary pulmonary hypertension, PH-SEC=pulmonary hypertension of a secondary nature, IPF= idiopathic pulmonary fibrosis, BRONCH= bronchiectasis, EMP=emphysema, EMP A-1=alpha-1 antitrypsin deficiency, LAM=lung AV malformation.

however, have reached the two year anniversary of transplantation.

Although only early and intermediate results are available at the present time on pediatric lung transplantation, comparison of the lung transplant results with the few reported series of heart-lung transplantation for pediatric patients suggests that the overall results can be expected to be comparable between these two types of treatments.[31-35] The indications for combined heart-lung transplantation rather than pulmonary transplantation remain unclear. Early results with cardiac repair and single or bilateral lung transplantation in patients with pulmonary hypertension and congenital heart disease have been acceptable and an increasing number of adults with intracardiac defects have now

undergone repair and single or bilateral sequential transplantation.[36,37] In addition, the technique of pulmonary transplantation and cardiac repair has been extended to those patients with more complex types of congenital defects requiring fairly elaborate repairs such as pulmonary atresia with ventricular septal defect and lack of central pulmonary arteries. Lung transplantation and cardiac repair has also been performed in adults with atrioventricular canal defects. The early measurement of pulmonary pressures and cardiac function have been encouraging in these patients, however, the long-term effects of correction of congenital heart defects on ventricular function and ventricular compliance is unknown. If these encouraging early results are maintained then it is possible that expansion of lung transplantation and cardiac repair to more complex forms of congenital heart disease including diagnoses such as transposition of the great arteries with VSD and Eisenmenger's syndrome may be possible. The advantage of cardiac repair and lung transplantation is the maximum utilization of scarce donor organs with the potential availability of the donor heart for use in an additional recipient. In these patients, a "domino" procedure would not be possible. Combined heart and lung transplantation will continue to have a major place in the transplantation armamentarium, especially for those children with significant left ventricular dysfunction accompanying their end-stage pulmonary disease.

Although it was hoped that bronchiolitis obliterans would be less common in patients undergoing pulmonary transplantation as opposed to those who have heart-lung transplantation, it is now evident that the incidence of bronchiolitis obliterans is not significantly different in these two techniques.[30,38–40] Bronchiolitis obliterans remains a significant complication of both single and bilateral lung transplantation and affects 25–40% of survivors.[30] Children may represent a particularly vulnerable group for the development of this complication since rejection and viral challenges may be more frequent in children than in adults, assuming that the underlying etiology for this is related to one of these two factors. Our approach to these patients with bronchiolitis obliterans is to augment their immunosuppression with a course of ATG and an increase in the cyclosporine and steroid doses. The overall effectiveness of this therapy has been reasonably good although it is much too early to draw any firm conclusions. Bronchiolitis obliterans remains the major obstacle to long-term success in lung transplantation.

CONCLUSIONS

From our results of pulmonary transplantation in children at St. Louis Children's Hospital and a review of the pediatric transplants reported to date along with the international results in the St. Louis Lung Transplant Registry, it is apparent that pulmonary transplantation can be performed in children with acceptable early results. As shown earlier, however, the majority of pediatric lung transplants have been performed for cystic fibrosis and relatively few pediatric patients have had transplants for Eisenmenger's syndrome, primary pulmonary hypertension or pulmonary fibrosis. The small experience in the pediatric age range coupled with a variation in indications for transplant make for difficult comparison with the adult population. In addition, pediatric pulmonary transplantation has only been performed relatively recently and long-term follow-up data are not available. The intermediate-term results suggest that the results are likely to be similar to those noted with heart-lung transplantation in children, for which there is a somewhat longer follow-up available. Whether pulmonary or heart-lung transplantation is the preferred technique in children, it is apparent that these patients represent a particularly difficult group and careful selection coupled with attention to multiple medical conditions relating to the underlying disease process are required for optimal results to be achieved. Finally, the combination of smaller patients and longer waiting times together promote expansion of the use of lobar or reduced-size transplants and living related lobar transplants for children. As experience with this technical refinement of lung transplantation grows we can expect to see higher risk infants considered for lung transplantation in what was formerly considered a hopeless situation.

REFERENCES

1. The Toronto Lung Transplant Group. Unilateral lung transplantation for pulmonary fibrosis. N Engl J Med 1986; 314:1140-5.
2. St. Louis International Lung Transplant Registry. Suite 3108 Queeny Tower, #1 Barnes Hospital Plaza, St. Louis, MO 63110.
3. Spray TL, Mallory GB, Canter CE, Huddleston CB, Kaiser LR. Pediatric lung transplantation for pulmonary hypertension and congenital heart disease. Ann Thorac Surg 1992; 54:216-25.

4. De Hoyos A, Maurer JR. Complications following lung transplantation. Semin Thorac Cardiovasc Surg 1992; 4:132-46.

5. Registry, Extracorporeal Life Support Organization, 1500 E. Medical Center Drive, Ann Arbor, MI 48109. November, 1992 report.

6. Cromblehome TM, Adzick NS, Hardy K et al. Pulmonary lobartransplantation in neonatal swine: a model for treatment of congenital diaphragmatic hernia. J Pediatr Surg 1990; 25:11-8.

7. Calhoon JH, Grover IL, Gibbons WJ et al. Single lung transplantation: alter-native indications and techniques. J Thorac Cardiovasc Surg 1991; 101:816-25.

8. Patterson GA. Airway complications. Chest Surg Clin N Am 1993; 3:157-73.

9. McKeown PP, Tsuboi H, Togo T et al. Growth of tracheal anastomoses: advantage of absorbable interrupted sutures. Ann Thorac Surg 1991; 51:636-41.

10. Spray TL, Huddleston CB. Pediatric lung transplantation. Chest Surg Clin N Am 1993; 3:123-43.

11. Dunnill MS. Postnatal growth of the lung. Thorax 1962; 17:329-33.

12. Davies G, Reid L. Growth of the alveoli and pulmonary arteries in childhood. Thorax 1970:25:669-81.

13. Thurlbeck WM. Postnatal human lung growth. Thorax 1982; 37:564-71.

14. Hislop AA, Odom NJ, McGregor CGA, Haworth SG. Growth potential of the immature transplanted lung: an experimental study. J Thorac Cardiovasc Surg 1990; 100:360-70.

15. Rinaldi M, Hislop A, Odom NJ, Haworth SG, McGregor CGA. Surgical factors affecting growth potential of the immature rat lung. Eur J Cardio-thorac Surg 1991; 5:218-22.

16. Haverich A, Dammenhayn L, Demertzis S et al. Lung growth after experimental pulmonary transplantation. J Heart Lung Transplant 1991; 10:288-95.

17. Kern JA, Tribble CG, Flanagan TL et al. Growth potential of porcine reduced-size mature pulmonary lobar transplants. J Thorac Cardiovasc Surg 1992; 104:1329-32.

18. Crombleholme TM, Adzick NS, Longaker MT et al. Reduced-size lung transplantation in neonatal swine: technique and short-term physiological response. Ann Thorac Surg 1990; 49:55-60.

19. Kern JA, Tribble CG, Chan BBK et al. Reduced-size porcine lung transplantation: long-term studies of pulmonary vascular resistance. Ann Thorac Surg 1992; 53:583-9.

20. Hislop AA, Wigglesworth JS, Desai R. Alveolar development in the human fetus and infant. Early human development 1986; 13:1-11.

21. Lillehei CW, Everts E, Shamberger RC. Reduced-size lung transplantation from adult to neonatal sheep. J Pediatr Surg 1992; 27:1153-6.

22. Backer CL, Ohtake S, Zales VR et al. Living related lobar lung transplantation in beagle puppies. J Pediatr Surg 1991; 26:429-33.

23. Jennings RW, Lorenz HP, Duncan BW et al. Adult-to-neonate lung transplantation: anatomic considerations. J Pediatr Surg 1992; 10:1285-90.

24. Kolata, G. Lungs from parents fail to save girl, 9, and doctors assess ethics. New York Times, May 20, 1991.

25. Starnes VA, Lewiston NJ, Luikart H et al. Current trends in lung transplantation: lobar transplantation and expanded use of single lungs. J Thorac Cardiovasc Surg 1992; 104:1060-6.

26. Laros CD, Westermann CJJ. Dilatation, compensatory growth, or both after pneumonectomy during childhood and adolescence: a thirty-year follow-up study. J Thorac Cardiovasc Surg 1987; 93:570-6.

27. Griffith BP, Hardesty RL, Armitage JM et al. Management of dysfunction in the transplanted lung: experience with seven clinical cases. Ann Thorac Surg 1992; 53:635-41.

28. Bolman, RM, Shumway SJ, Braunlin, E et al. Pediatric lung and heart-lung transplantation. J Heart-Lung Transplant 1991; 10:162.

29. Miller JD, Patterson GA. Retransplantation following isolated lung transplantation. Semin Cardiovasc Surg 1992; 4:122-5.

30. M'etras D, Shennib H, Kreitmann B, Camboulives J et al. Double-lung transplantation in children: a report of 20 cases.

Ann Thorac Surg 1993; 55:352-7.

31. Michler RE, Rose EA. Pediatric heart and heart-lung transplantation. Ann Thorac Surg 1991; 52:708-9.

32. Smyth RL, Scott JP, Whitehead B et al. The use of heart-lung transplantation in management of terminal respiratory complications of cystic fibrosis. Transplant Proc 1990; 22:1472-3.

33. Smyth RL, Scott JP, Whitehead B et al. Heart-lung transplantation in children. Transplant Proc 1990; 22:1470-1.

34. Starnes VA, Marshall SE, Lewiston NJ et al. Heart-lung transplantation in infants, children, and adolescents. J Pediatr Surg 1991; 26:434-8.

35. Armitage JM, Kormos RL, Flicker FJ. Pediatric pulmonary transplantation: the University of Pittsburgh experience. J Heart-Lung Transplant 1991; 10:162.

36. Fremes SE, Patterson GA, Williams WG et al. Single lung transplantation and closure of patent ductus arteriosus for Eisenmenger's Syndrome. J Thorac Cardiovasc Surg 1990; 100:1-5.

37. Bove E. Lung transplantation and repairs of congenital heart defects. Presented at American Academy of Pediatrics. San Francisco, CA, Sept, 1992.

38. Maurer JR, Morrison D, Winton TL et al. Late pulmonary complications of isolated lung transplantation. Transplant Proc 1991; 23:1224-5.

39. Scott JP, Sharples L, Mullins P et al. Further studies on the natural history of obliterative bronchiolitis following heart-lung transplantation. Transplant Proc 191; 23:1201-2.

40. Starnes VA, Lewiston N, Theodore J et al. Cystic fibrosis: target population for lung transplantation in North America in the 1990s. J Thorac Cardiovasc Surg 1992; 103:1008-14.

CHAPTER 3

PRESERVATION OF THE REDUCED-SIZE LUNG ALLOGRAFT

Charles D. Fraser, Jr.
William A. Baumgartner

INTRODUCTION

Successful clinical application of lung transplantation was introduced by Reitz and associates who first reported the use of combined cardiopulmonary transplantation in 1981.[1] The pioneering work of Cooper and colleagues demonstrated the applicability of single and double-lung transplantation in patients with pulmonary fibrosis and end-stage pulmonary vascular disease.[2-4] These promising results in the adult population led to expansion of lung transplantation techniques to children with pulmonary hypertension associated with correctable congenital heart defects.[5-7]

Despite these advances, the field of lung transplantation, especially in children, has not experienced the growth that heart transplantation has.[8] Donor organ availability continues to be a prime factor limiting increased application of this technique. This fact has prompted investigation into the use of reduced-size (lobar) pulmonary allografts either from living related or cadaveric donors.[7,9-12] Initial clinical success has been encouraging and has demonstrated that the potential donor pool can be expanded by the procurement of multiple organs from one cadaveric donor and by adding the option of living related donation.[13]

Reduced-size Lung Transplantation, edited by John A. Kern, M.D. and Irving L. Kron, M.D.; © 1993 R.G. Landes Company.

Ex vivo organ preservation continues to be another factor limiting the donor pool. Techniques for lung preservation that have been used clinically to date have provided satisfactory preservation for up to six hours of ischemia.[14-16] Despite acceptable results, however, early graft dysfunction still occurs, presumably as the result of inadequate preservation.[17] In addition, most centers will not accept organs for donation which will require ischemic intervals beyond the four to six hour time limit. This results in suboptimal donor organ distribution and recipient matching.

There is considerable disparity between what has been demonstrated in the research laboratory in terms of pulmonary preservation and what is applied clinically. Most lung transplant surgeons today rely on some form of hypothermic pulmonary flush solution (usually crystalloid) followed by static, topical cold preservation. These methods of preservation have been preferred for their simplicity and reproducibility.[16-18] There is clearly sufficient data in the literature to suggest that further refinements and modification of currently used techniques could improve organ preservation and lengthen acceptable ischemic intervals.

In this chapter, the topic of pulmonary preservation for transplantation will be reviewed. Emphasis will be placed on the current understanding of mechanisms of pulmonary ischemic injury as well as neurohumoral alterations occurring in the transplanted lung. Experimental data investigating interventions designed to address these mechanisms of lung injury will be reviewed. Where appropriate, particular attention will be directed toward issues of pulmonary preservation peculiar to the reduced-size lung allograft. Finally, currently used clinical lung preservation techniques will be summarized.

ISCHEMIC LUNG INJURY

Due to its unique delicate anatomical structure, the lung is more sensitive to the effects of ischemia, reperfusion and manipulation when compared to other organs. The lung's response to ischemia is similar in many ways to the response seen with other pathologic insults including endotoxemia, hyperoxia and inhalation of toxic gases. The ultimate physiologic manifestation of injury is derived from a complex interaction within both the lung itself and circulating humoral and cellular blood elements.[19]

The final pathophysiologic manifestation of ischemic lung injury as the result of inadequate preservation may be detected as an abnormal increase in interstitial lung water. As the alveolar-capillary membrane barrier is damaged, the pulmonary interstitium takes on excess water. The composition of this fluid is different from that of cardiogenic pulmonary edema in that it is exudative as opposed to transudative. Due to the increased protein content of this fluid, pulmonary edema results at lower critical hydrostatic pressures than in edema of cardiac causes. The amount of extravascular lung water correlates with other measurements of lung function, including diminished airway compliance, impaired gas exchange and increased pulmonary vascular resistance.[21]

The histopathologic changes associated with an acute ischemic pulmonary insult include alveolar and interstitial edema, alveolar-capillary membrane disruption and hemorrhage. These changes may be diffuse or patchy, and relatively normal areas of lung tissue may be located adjacent to areas of severe injury. Section of pulmonary capillaries may reveal leukocyte and platelet trapping. Standard chest radiographs demonstrate a spectrum of changes ranging from mild interstitial edema to complete opacification. These changes are typical of the reimplantation response after lung transplantation as described by Siegelman in 1973 and are now known to represent macroscopic evidence of the ischemia-reperfusion injury phenomenon.[22,23]

The duration of warm ischemia that the lung can tolerate is not entirely clear and may depend, in part, on whether or not the lung is ventilated. Early studies by Blades and later by Egan have documented that ventilated lungs subjected to as much as four hours of warm ischemia maintain gas exchange function.[24,25] Stevens et al, Fonkulsrud et al, and more recently, Puskas and associates, have each observed enhanced lung tolerance to ischemia in dogs subjected to hyperventilation prior to the ischemic period.[26-28] It is unclear whether this observation is related to the beneficial effect of hyperinflation on pulmonary surfactant release from type II pneumonocytes or by the provision of oxygen substrate for aerobic metabolism during ischemia. The act of hyperinflation may be the important feature, however, while the addition of oxygen may actually be harmful as observed by Fisher et al. They studied ischemic rat lungs ventilated with varying concentrations of oxygen and observed increased lipid peroxidation as measured by thiobarbituric acid reactive products and conjugated dienes in those animals receiving higher concentrations.[29] The issue of donor lung hyperinflation will be discussed in more detail in a later section.

The physiologic mechanism of the ischemia-reperfusion insult has been the subject of considerable investigation and appears to occur largely at the subcellular level. Numerous studies have demonstrated that the restoration of blood flow to ischemic tissues causes increased microvascular leakage of plasma proteins, solutes and water. The endothelial cell damage is due to the generation of toxic oxygen-derived free radicals. This has been observed in a variety of species and in multiple organ models.[30-32]

Endothelial cell damage is initiated at the cell membrane level by free radical induced lipid peroxidation. Oxygen-derived free radical species, which possess single unpaired electrons, are produced during normal mitochondrial respiration by the reduction of molecular oxygen that generates superoxide anions (O_2^-), and hydroxyl radicals (OH^-). The hydroxyl radical is highly reactive and interacts with a wide variety of molecules, yielding unstable products capable of causing further adverse reactions. The cell's natural defense against this process includes several important enzymes including superoxide dismutase (SOD) and vitamin E which play important roles in protection against oxidation of membrane phospholipids.[33,34] During ischemia the balance between free radical production and removal is shifted toward radical accumulation. One principal mechanism is

through the production of xanthine oxidase (XO) which catalyzes the reaction of hypoxanthine with oxygen producing xanthine and superoxide radicals. The hypoxanthine substrate accumulates in ischemic tissues as the result of adenosine triphosphate catabolism. Reperfusion provides molecular oxygen for the catabolism of hypoxanthine, resulting in the formation of further free radicals. Under normal physiologic conditions, SOD can remove the majority of O_2^-. In the presence of molecular iron (Fe^{3+}), the excess O_2^- can be converted to OH^- via the Haber-Weiss reaction.[35] This reactive hydroxyl radical causes lipid peroxidation by extracting a hydrogen atom from polyunsaturated fatty acids, generating a lipid alkyl radical. A molecular rearrangement of the double bonds then takes place forming diene conjugates. Oxygen can then react to create peroxy radicals that can propagate the process (Figs. 1,2).

The intracellular concentration of Ca^{++} is closely regulated and Ca^{++} entry into the cell is via specific receptor-operated channels. It is extruded from the cells by a Na^+/Ca^{++} exchange mechanism and by active transport. If this situation becomes deranged, elevated Ca^{++} levels in the cytosol result in increased conversion of xanthine dehydrogenase to XO. Another important consequence of elevated Ca^{++} is the activation of membrane phospholipases which act on membrane phospholipids to further destabilize the cell membrane.[36] Arachidonic acid that is removed from the cell membrane is a substrate for cyclooxygenase that catalyzes a reaction yielding prostaglandin H_2 which is then converted to several other products including thromboxane (vasoconstrictor) and prostacyclin (vasodilator). During ischemia the accumulation of peroxides, which inhibit the formation of prostacyclin, shift the balance in favor of vasoconstriction. Via the lipoxygenase pathway arachidonic acid is also the substrate for the production of leukotrienes, substances that cause potent vaso- and bronchoconstriction.[37]

The presence of neutrophils in the microvasculature at the time of reperfusion is known to play an important role in this oxidant mediated response, however, the degree

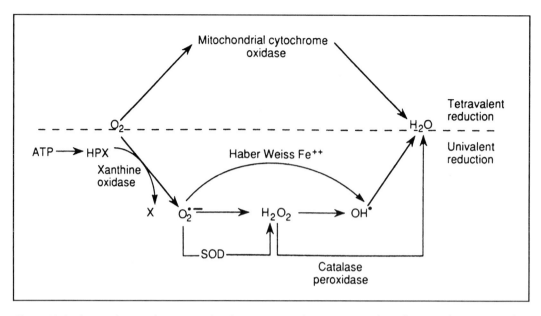

Fig. 1. Univalent pathway of oxygen reduction. Hypoxanthine (HPX) and xanthine oxidase accumulate in stored tissues. At the time of reperfusion, O_2^- (superoxide). Superoxide can then be converted to hydroxyl by the Haber-Weiss reaction.

of their contribution is not agreed upon. Adkins et al evaluated the effect of ischemia-reperfusion on pulmonary capillary permeability in isolated rabbit lungs and the roles of XO, aldehyde oxidase (AO) and neutrophils (PMN) in producing lung injury.[38] Inactivation of AO had no effect in attenuating the increase in pulmonary vascular permeability seen after reperfusion. XO inhibition by allopurinol and prevention of PMN endothelial adhesion by the monoclonal antibody IB_4 were both successful in ameliorating the ischemia-induced changes in endothelial permeability. They concluded that an interaction between XO and PMN is necessary to cause the lung damage associated with ischemia-reperfusion since inhibiting either prevented the increased permeability. The proposed

$$O_2^{\cdot -} + Fe^{3+} \rightarrow Fe^{2+} + O_2$$

$$2\, O_2^{\cdot -} + 2\, H^+ \rightarrow H_2O_2 + O_2$$

$$Fe^{2+} + H_2O_2 \rightarrow Fe^{3+} + OH^- + OH\cdot$$

Fig. 2. Haber-Weiss reaction for conversion of superoxide to hydroxyl in the presence of molecular iron.

mechanism involves the production of super-oxide radical by XO, which in addition to causing endothelial cell damage, serves as a chemotactic agent and activator of neutrophil activity. The resultant action of the activated PMN including release of lysozymal enzymes augments endothelial injury. Similar studies from others have also supported the role of the PMN in this response.[31,39] The overall process is not yet fully elucidated but likely is a continuum involved superoxide

generation and PMN augmentation of the response. As mentioned previously, the presence of oxygen in hyperinflated ischemic lungs has been observed to result in increased lipid peroxidation. This was observed to occur in the absence of circulating PMN as the lungs were studied in an isolated preparation and were perfused with an acellular, synthetic perfusate.[29] Presumably, resident pulmonary leukocytes could have played some role in this response (Fig. 3).

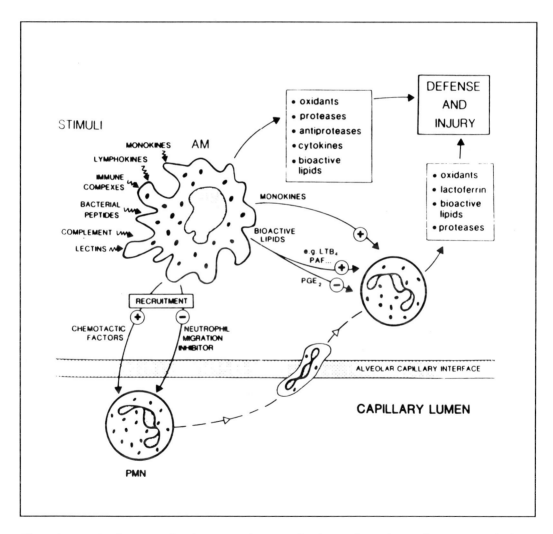

Fig. 3. Interaction between alveolar macrophages and polymorphonuclear cells (PMNs) in the lung. Alveolar macrophages release chemotatic factors for PMN. Once in the alveolar lumen, PMNs can be activated by various factors to influence the injury process.

In summary, ischemia induced lung injury is the result of abnormal pulmonary capillary permeability caused by a constellation of molecular events including oxygen-derived radical lipid peroxidation. PMNs act to augment this process, resulting in a cascade of events resulting in endothelial damage. Increased interstitial and alveolar fluid results in diminished airway compliance, increased vascular resistance, hemorrhage and impaired gas exchange.

PULMONARY PRESERVATION

HYPOTHERMIA

All methods of lung preservation that are being used clinically today rely on deep hypothermia. As an interesting historical note, however, early efforts at lung preservation for transplantation involved the use of the autoperfused, normothermic working heart-lung preparation for distant procurements. This concept was first described by Martin in 1883 and later was used by Starling in his classic experiments.[40,41] Robicsek and associates demonstrated the utility of the autoperfusion concept as a means of providing extracorporeal preservation of the heart.[42] Griffith and colleagues successfully applied this technique to clinical heart-lung transplantation at the University of Pittsburgh. The technique has since been abandoned, however, as more simple, static hypothermic methods have been developed.[43]

The fact that cold, static pulmonary protection provides adequate preservation for transplantation was demonstrated by Cooper and associates in their important papers relating their initial clinical experience with unilateral lung transplantation.[2,3] In these reports the authors simply immersed the explanted pulmonary grafts uninflated in cold (4°C) crystalloid solution of intracellular composition (Collins solution). This simple technique was successful in providing satisfactory preservation for up to 5.5 hours of donor organ ischemia.

The use of pulmonary graft hypothermia for preservation had its origin in other fields

of solid organ transplantation. The observation that simple topical hypothermia provides adequate myocardial protection for transplantation was demonstrated by Shumway and colleagues in their landmark work in heart transplantation done at Stanford University.[44] Organ cooling reduces metabolic demand and thereby, adenosine triphosphate utilization. Cellular metabolism is slowed and cell membrane integrity is maintained through avoidance of the above mentioned cascade of events of ischemia-reperfusion. This simple technique, however, has definite time limitations as even at low temperatures some cellular energy metabolism must continue to maintain membrane integrity and intracellular-extracellular ionic gradients. These conditions apply to pulmonary preservation as well.

It is particularly interesting to note that there is some considerable disagreement regarding the optimal organ temperature for hypothermic preservation. Wang and associates demonstrated that in an isolated perfused rabbit lung model, pulmonary preservation at 10°C provided superior protection when compared to lungs preserved at 4°C.[45] Despite such data, however, most transplant surgeons still prefer to keep lung grafts as cold as possible without inducing crystal formation. This usually translates into storage media temperatures of around 4°C.

The optimal technique for cooling the pulmonary graft is also the subject of some debate. Basically, aside from simple immersion there are two techniques that have been used to provide cooling of the lung parenchyma. One involves some form of hypothermic pulmonary artery flush, either a synthetic intracellular or extracellular solution, or cooling of the entire donor and thereby, the lungs, using deep systemic hypothermia on cardiopulmonary bypass.

At the Johns Hopkins Hospital, we have conducted experimental investigation evaluating the efficacy of donor core-cooling as a means of providing deep hypothermic protection of the pulmonary graft. In small dairy calves, we have observed excellent pulmonary preservation for ischemic times up to six hours without substrate enhancement or pulmonary flushing. In comparing donor core-cooling to standard pulmonary flush techniques (Euro-Collins at 4°C) we observed improved donor lung function as determined by gas exchange, lung compliance, extravascular lung water and histology.[46,47] Because of these laboratory studies, we have used donor core-cooling clinically as our preferred preservation technique since 1983. With this method, we have achieved satisfactory pulmonary preservation for ischemic times up to 5.5 hours.[48]

The core-cooling technique basically involves placing the donor on cardiopulmonary bypass using a portable unit developed by the perfusion service at Johns Hopkins. The technique allows for gradual yet thorough cooling of the entire donor, and therefore, all organs for harvest without the necessity of flushing. The technique also allows for consistent blood pressure control, avoiding the rapid changes often observed during dissection of donor organs prior to harvest. Once a core temperature of 10–15°C is reached, the donor is exsanguinated into the bypass reservoir. At this time, harvest can proceed as per usual in a near bloodless field with all organs already being cooled. The technique, of course, does not preclude flushing, as many groups have concerns regarding residual blood and PMNs in the lung graft. We have not flushed the grafts and have observed satisfactory function (Fig. 4).

The core-cooling technique has not been used for harvest of a reduced-size lung graft, however, this method would seem ideal for such a harvest in which a lobe was to be harvested from a lung block in a cadaveric donor. This technique allows uniform cooling of the lung graft without manipulation of the pulmonary vasculature.

Because of the somewhat cumbersome nature of transporting the bypass circuit as well as concerns over possible graft injury as a direct result of the potential inflammatory response initiated by bypass, most groups performing lung transplants have preferred the more simple cold flush technique.

As mentioned previously, the optimal temperature for hypothermic pulmonary preservation remains unclear. Similarly, the optimal perfusate temperature during cooling is also unclear.[45] The principal goal remains to provide thorough uniform cooling, and thereby, to reversibly inhibit the lung graft's metabolic function such that cell injury does not occur. In previous investigations simple topical cooling has been shown to be an inefficient method for lung cooling.[24,49] Especially with large lung grafts, uniform cooling is difficult to obtain by immersion, resulting in lengthened periods of warm ischemia. This problem may be somewhat obviated in a reduced-size allograft, although unpredictability of cooling should still be expected.

There are several theoretical advantages of hypothermic flush preservation of the lungs. The most obvious is the ability to provide rapid graft cooling. Many surgeons also feel very strongly that it is of great importance to flush out as much residual donor blood from the pulmonary vasculature as possible, and thusly, to prevent microvascular occlusion and endothelial injury from activated blood elements. As mentioned above, our experience with donor core-cooling would indicate that residual pulmonary vasculature blood may not be a significant problem. Of particular note is the fact that in a review of all research into flush perfusion methods for the lung, no one technique has been shown to provide consistently predictable results.[18]

An interesting laboratory study has recently been published by Cooper and colleagues evaluating methods of cold flushing and topical cooling and the effect of temperature of the flushing solution on lung preservation.[50] In an ex vivo rabbit lung model, they demonstrated that flushing with a phosphate-buffered dextran solution provided superior preservation when compared to simple topical cooling by immersion. Of more interest was their observation that flushing with room temperature (23°C) perfusate and subsequent storage at 10°C provided superior postischemic function compared to flushing at 10°C and cold storage. The reasons for

their findings are not entirely clear but may
relate to similar observations in other organ
systems.[51,52] Rapid flushing of the lungs at

very low temperatures may have several
deleterious effects. Even with administration
of vasodilators cold flushing may cause intense

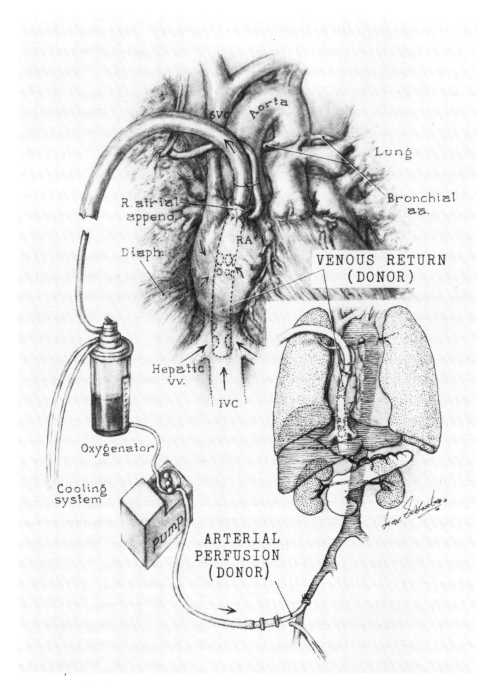

Fig. 4. Portable donor core-cooling system for hypothermic pulmonary preservation.

vasoconstriction. The increased vascular resistance may result in incomplete and inhomogeneous cooling. It also could contribute to incomplete blood washout. In animals flushed with perfusate at 23°C the authors observed lower pulmonary vascular resistance, thus supporting the hypothesis that vasoconstriction is avoided, providing more complete flushing. They have theorized that perhaps the most efficacious method would involve flushing the lungs with perfusate of gradually decreasing temperature down to 10°C. They feel that the optimal storage temperature is around 10°C as demonstrated in their earlier studies.[49]

PULMONARY FLUSH COMPOSITION

As with preservation temperature there is no consensus of opinion as to what constitutes the optimal pulmonary flush solution. Considerable research has been done in this area with the goal being to provide uniform cooling, pulmonary vasodilation and maintain cellular integrity and function.

An area of intense investigation has centered on the question of whether superior preservation is provided by solutions of intra- or extracellular composition. Solutions with ionic compositions similar to extracellular fluid, especially normal saline, have previously been shown to be ineffective, resulting in considerable cellular edema and loss of endothelial integrity.[18] These findings led investigation into the development of hyperosmolar solutions designed to prevent intracellular edema. Since 1984 modified Euro-Collins solution (EC) has been the most commonly used flush solution for clinical lung transplantation. Initial experimental and clinical reports indicated that cold EC could be used to provide satisfactory pulmonary preservation for ischemic intervals of up to eight hours.[14,17,53] Despite our findings that donor core-cooling provided superior organ function after transplantation when compared to the EC, the simple EC flush method has been the most widely accepted. Nonetheless, clinical experience has now shown that organ preservation after EC flush is unpredictable, with varying degrees of organ dysfunction after transplantation being demonstrated.[54]

The University of Wisconsin(UW) solution was developed in 1986 and is now the flush solution of choice for clinical hepatic and renal transplantation.[55-57] These results have prompted significant experimental and clinical investigation of UW solution as a pulmonary flush solution for transplantation. Unruh has evaluated the vascular and interstitial effects of UW flush in the canine lung.[58] He observed a slight increase in vascular tone but no change in wet-dry ratios, interstitial compliance and transvascular fluid flux. His final conclusion was that UW did not cause pulmonary edema in this model (Table 1).

In comparing EC and UW in a rat lung preservation model, Semik and associates have demonstrated superior postpreservation oxygenation, wet-dry ratios, pulmonary vascular resistance and compliance in lungs receiving UW.[59] Others have demonstrated similar encouraging results using UW solution for pulmonary flush.[60,61] Griffith and associates have recently published their clinical results retrospectively comparing EC with UW in patients undergoing either single lung, double lung or heart-lung transplantation.[62] They observed increased reperfusion injury as determined by postoperative chest radiography (day one) in the EC group when compared to the UW group despite the fact that the UW group had significantly longer ischemic times. Other measures of organ preservation studied, including alveolar-arterial oxygen gradients, length of postoperative intubation and early survival, were similar in the two groups. These results have led them to conclude that UW solution is at least as effective as EC for lung preservation, and perhaps better, due to the longer ischemic times in the UW group.

The beneficial effects of UW solution are believed to be derived from several factors. The hypertonic composition of UW is felt to prevent intracellular edema during cold ischemia. Although hypothermia plays a central role in lowering metabolic demands during preservation, it may act to promote

Table 1. Composition Of Euro-Collins (EC) And University Of Wisconsin (UW) Preservation Solutions.

Component	EC	UW
Potassium (mmol/L)	107	125
Sodium (mmol/L)	9.3	30
Magnesium (mmol/L)	4.7	5
Chloride (mmol/L)	14	—
Bicarbonate (mmol/L)	9.3	—
Phosphate (mmol/L)	55	25
Sulfate (mmol/L)	4.7	5
Lactobionate (mmol/L)	—	100
Raffinose (mmol/L)	—	30
Glutathione (mmol/L)	—	3
Adenosine (mmol/L)	—	5
Allopurinol (mmol/L)	—	1
Glucose (%)	5.6	—
Mannitol (%)	0.58	—
Hydroxyethyl starch (%)	—	5.0
Insulin (U/L)	—	100
Dexamethasone (mg/L)	—	8
pH	7.74	7.87
Osmolality (mOsm/L)	452	327

cellular swelling by inhibiting the membrane bound Na^+/K^+ pump, thus, allowing for an influx of Na^+ and water into the cells. Lactobionate, raffinose and hydroxyethyl starch act extracellularly to increase osmotic pressure. Glutathione and allopurinol act as antioxidants and adenosine is known to be a potent pulmonary vasodilator. This results in more even cooling of the lung graft.

Low potassium-dextran solution (LPD) is another solution that has been studied in providing pulmonary flush preservation. Although the solution is of extracellular composition, the addition of the impermeant Dextran-40 (hydroxyethyl starch 20 gm/l) presumably adds the beneficial effect of preventing cellular edema. Steen and associates studied porcine lung allografts perfused with LPD and subjected to 12 hours of hypothermic (4°C) preservation.[63] They observed adequate pulmonary preservation in this model as determined by acute animal survival and arterial oxygen tension. These authors stressed the importance of a low potassium concentration in the perfusate (4 mEq/l for LPD versus 108 mEq/l for EC and 125 mEq/l for UW) in preventing pulmonary vasoconstriction. They also emphasized their opinion that prevention of atelectasis during perfusion is critical in avoiding incomplete and inhomogeneous cooling. Other reports in the literature have provided conflicting results, demonstrating equivalent[64] or superior[65] hypothermic protection of the lung graft.

It should be mentioned that some groups, most notably the group at Papworth Hospital, have advocated the use of cold modified blood to perfuse the pulmonary graft. A study by Hooper et al[66] in 1990 has demonstrated that in a canine model EC solution provides superior preservation as assessed by pulmonary vascular resistance, compliance and lung water determination.

Unfortunately, the wide variety of experimental models, as well as differences in technique, make interpretation of differences in perfusion solutions somewhat difficult. It would appear, however, that an important feature of the "ideal" solution is a cell membrane impermeable substance to prevent cell edema formation. In addition, solutions with high potassium concentrations likely induce significant pulmonary vasospasm and thusly result in suboptimal cooling.

ROLE OF PROSTAGLANDINS IN LUNG PRESERVATION

Prostaglandins are products of arachidonic acid metabolism that have a wide variety of biologic effects. Prostaglandin E_1 (PGE_1) and prostacyclin (PGI_2) have received particular attention in lung preservation research due their potent properties as pulmonary vasodilators.[67] These agents are also bronchodilators and have been observed to have a variety of protective effects on the lung subjected to various insults including warm ischemia.[68] Prostaglandins have been shown to have cytoprotective effects, thought to be related to properties of stabilization of

lysosomal membranes.[69] They also are known to attenuate leukocyte sequestration and platelet aggregation and thus limit tissue damage in situations in which injury may be augmented by leukocyte adhesion and activation.[70] They may also have a role in limiting increases in vascular permeability initiated by inflammatory mediators.

Both PGE_1 and PGI_2 have been used clinically as adjuncts to pulmonary artery flush methods for lung preservation. As with other aspects of lung preservation, there is considerable disagreement in the literature as to which agent has the greatest efficacy in improving pulmonary preservation.

Since the initial reports by the Stanford group of successful static lung preservation after donor pretreatment with PGE_1 followed by cold EC flush, many groups have adopted PGE_1 infusion as part of their lung procurement protocols.[71,72] As noted above, PGE_1 is a potent vasodilator and it has been used in lung flush techniques to ameliorate the known vasoconstrictor effects of cold EC. Despite its widespread clinical use, however, it is notable that several recent laboratory investigations have cast doubt on the true efficacy of PGE_1 in lung preservation. In studies by Bonser and colleagues, donor pretreatment with PGE_1 was noted to have deleterious effects on lung preservation in a canine model of transplantation after 12 hours preservation.[73,74] In an isolated rabbit lung preservation model, graft treatment with PGE_1 did not improve the performance of low potassium-dextran as a flush solution. These authors observed no improvement in lungs preserved with PGE_1 and LPD flush versus LPD alone.[75] In a study of canine single lung transplantation, Novick and associates compared lungs preserved with cold EC flush after pretreatment with either saline, PGE_1 or PGI_2. They observed superior graft function after PGI_2 treatment, while treatment with PGE_1 conferred no apparent benefit.[76] They hypothesize that this observed difference must be related to some effect of PGI_2 other that vasodilation, an effect also provided by PGE_1. The authors note that the lungs are a major site for the synthesis, release and degradation of most prostaglandins, including PGE_1. Prostacyclin, however, is not inactivated by the lung but is hydrolyzed to a more stable metabolite in the liver. In addition, PGI_2 is known to be a more potent inhibitor of platelet aggregation.[77,78]

Considerable experimental and clinical evidence exists that indicates a beneficial role of PGI_2 in lung preservation. Mulvin and colleagues investigated the role of the vasodilator properties of PGI_2 in a rat lung preservation model.[79] They demonstrated improved lung preservation as reflected in diminished wet gain in lungs flushed with a solution containing prostacyclin. They also noted, however, that a similar effect could be achieved by donor treatment with a nitroglycerine infusion, thus leading them to conclude that the protective effect of PGI_2 was predominantly due to its vasodilator properties.

As noted above, Novick and associates have documented superior lung preservation after 12 hours of ischemia in grafts pretreated with PGI_2 infusion prior to harvest.[76] Prostacyclin was infused into donor dogs at an initial rate of 0.1 microgram/kg/min and the dose was titrated to reduce systemic arterial pressure by 40%. The lungs were then flushed with cold (4°C) EC. The authors have postulated that the improved preservation observed in their model with PGI_2 may be the result of other properties aside from vasodilation as PGE_1 was also given in a dose sufficient to reduce systemic blood pressure by 40%. They theorize that other potent effects of PGI_2 on platelet aggregation, leukocyte adhesion and membrane stability may explain the observe difference in their model. These promising results have been supported by other experimental studies.[80]

A very interesting study evaluating bronchial perfusion in pigs undergoing unilateral lung transplantation has demonstrated another potential beneficial effect of PGI_2. In this study Haverich and colleagues documented increased bronchial mucosal blood flow in lungs in which both donor and recipients received PGI_2 infusion.[81] This study has obvious clinical implications for the use of prostaglandin to improve bronchial anastomotic healing.

Clearly, prostaglandins play a central role in successful pulmonary preservation involving lengthy ischemic times. Whether PGE_1 or PGI_2 is most efficacious is not entirely clear. The above mentioned experimental evidence would indicate that PGI_2 may provide other beneficial effects aside from pulmonary vasodilation. At present PGE_1 is more commonly used, however. In terms of lung preservation in the reduced size graft, some form of prostaglandin use should be a part of the preservation protocol. Obviously, in the living related donor situation the systemic administration of prostaglandin is inadvisable due to the risk of profound systemic hypotension. In these situations, the lung flush solution should contain prostaglandin to be infused after the graft has been removed from the donor.

EFFECT OF VENTILATION ON PRESERVATION

As noted in the section on ischemic lung injury, considerable research has been done in evaluating the role of lung inflation during ischemic preservation.[25-28] In the canine lung transplant model Puskas and associates have documented satisfactory acute lung graft function after 30 hours of hypothermic ischemic preservation.[28] Donor lungs in this experiment were hyperinflated prior to harvest and then were flushed with cold EC with or without pretreatment with PGE_1. The transplanted lungs from the hyperinflated group demonstrated vastly superior function. The addition of PGE_1 to the preservation protocol conferred no additional benefit. In striking contrast, lungs harvested and stored in a semi-inflated state had uniformly poor function even with the addition of PGE_1. The authors in this important paper have hypothesized that the hyperinflation exerts its beneficial effect by allowing a more efficacious pulmonary artery flush as a result of avoidance of pulmonary vasoconstriction and atelectasis. They also note that hyperinflation has the additional effect of stimulating surfactant release, thereby preventing damaging alveolar collapse during storage.

Another interesting study that has indirectly demonstrated the importance of avoidance of atelectasis was performed by Klepetko and colleagues.[82] In a canine lung allotransplantation model they studied pulmonary surfactant levels as measured by levels of dipalmitoyl-phosphatidylcholine which is the main phosphocholine fraction of surfactant in bronchoalveolar lavage. In donor lungs pretreated with L-carnitine (an essential cofactor for transfer of long-chain fatty acids into the mitochondria), these investigators observed higher levels of pulmonary surfactant and improved postischemic lung function as determined by arterial oxygenation.

These important laboratory investigations strongly suggest that donor lung inflation is critical in organ preservation in which significant duration of ischemia is expected. As will be discussed later, there are considerable differences in practice at various lung transplant centers with regard to levels of lung inflation desired at the time of harvest. In the reduced-size graft, providing maximal inflation may be a difficult task unless the graft is taken from a larger, cadaveric donor in which the lung organ block is stored as the larger unit. This fact may be important in determining acceptable lengths of ischemia for the reduced size graft.

LEUKOCYTE DEPLETION AND LUNG PRESERVATION

Leukocytes, principally PMNs, are sequestered in ischemic lung tissues and are known to play a significant role in augmenting the reperfusion injury initiated by oxygen derived free radical species. Previous experimental investigation has determined that PMNs are intimately involved in mediating the endothelial injury observed in lung ischemia-reperfusion. Suzuki and colleagues have documented that blocking neutrophil adhesion to the vascular endothelium with monoclonal antibody prevents the enhanced permeability seen in reperfusion injury.[83]

Other in vitro studies have suggested that the ischemia-reperfusion lung injury may be ameliorated by leukocyte depletion.[84] These studies prompted further investigation in large animal models of lung transplantation. In a model of bovine double-lung transplantation, Schueler et al examined the effect of leukocyte depletion in donors and recipients on the ischemic tolerance of the transplanted lungs.[85] Donor lungs were preserved by donor core-cooling (no flush) on cardiopulmonary bypass. The bypass circuit was modified by the introduction of a mechanical filter that effectively reduced circulating leukocyte levels. The leukocyte filters were also employed in the bypass circuits used during the recipient implantation. Donor lungs harvested after leukocyte depletion and subjected to 24 hours of cold preservation demonstrated superior acute function when compared to lungs of nonleukocyte depleted recipients. This study confirmed previous reports by the same group utilizing shorter ischemic times.[86]

To date, no clinical studies have been done evaluating the effect of leukocyte depletion in lung transplantation. Clearly, effective leukocyte depletion depends on the use of cardiopulmonary bypass, which is often not used for clinical lung transplantation. This technique might prove applicable, however, in the use of reduced-size pulmonary allografts for lung transplantation in children who require simultaneous correction of congenital heart defects. Mechanical leukocyte filters placed in the bypass circuit are very effective in reducing circulating leukocyte counts for a short period after reperfusion. Presumably, this could be effective in minimizing the reperfusion injury.

MODULATION OF OXIDANT-INDUCED LUNG INJURY

As noted numerous times in other sections, oxygen-derived free radical species play a central role in ischemic lung injury, and consequently considerable research has been done in attempting to prevent or ameliorate this effect. Multiple studies have been done evaluating the effects of free radical scavengers in preserving lung function. In a rabbit lung transplant model, Alba and associates evaluated the effect of allopurinol on lung function after 6 hours of cold storage.[87] Allopurinol is an inhibitor of xanthine oxidase and is a hydroxyl radical scavenger. In this study, addition of allopurinol to the lung flush or the reperfusate resulted in improved lung function after cold ischemic storage. This study and others have strongly suggested that the addition of allopurinol to lung preservation solutions may be of significant benefit.[88,89] This may in part explain the clinically observed effectiveness of the University of Wisconsin solution in lung preservation.

Superoxide dismutase (SOD) is a naturally occurring free radical scavenger that is overwhelmed in the face of massive radical generation at the time of significant ischemia-reperfusion injury. The addition of SOD to flush solutions and to reperfusates has been shown to provide benefit in reducing reperfusion lung injury in some animal models.[68,90] This effect has not been achieved clinically, however, in part due to the large quantities of SOD that would be required to potentially be effective.

Calcium and iron play an important role in the univalent pathway of oxygen reduction (see above). Fe^{3+} reacts with oxygen radicals to generate toxic hydroxyl radicals. Desferrioxamine is an iron chelator and has been shown to be effective in animal models in radical induced lipid peroxidation. In the same experiment, addition of the calcium-channel blocker verapamil to the lung flush solution was also effective in reducing lipid peroxidation. Increases in cytosolic Ca^{2+} are known to augment the conversion of xanthine dehydrogenase to xanthine oxidase.[91] Potentially, the addition of either or both of these agents to lung flush solutions could be of significant clinical benefit. This matter merits further clinical investigation.

Lazaroids are a class of 21-aminosteroids. Several reports have reported these agents to be potent inhibitors of lipid peroxidation.[92] Aeba and associates have evaluated the effect of the lazaroid U74500A on lung preservation in an orthotopic rat lung transplant model. The addition of the lazaroid to the lung flush solution results in improved postischemic lung function and diminished lipid peroxidation as compared to a similar flush containing dexamethasone instead of lazaroid.[93] This study confirmed a previous investigation in a canine myocardial ischemia model.[94]

A variety of other agents have been studied in an effort to ameliorate oxidant-induced lung injury. Platelet activating factor (PAF) is a potent phospholipid mediator release by leukocytes, platelets and endothelial cells in response to several stimuli including ischemia-reperfusion.[95] PAF is thought to augment free radical induced lung injury by promoting the synthesis of arachidonic acid metabolites and through the oxygen burst phenomenon from phagocytic cells. In a recent canine lung preservation study, Wallace and associates demonstrated improved lung function after 6 hours of cold ischemia by pretreating donors and recipients with a PAF antagonist BN 52021.[96]

In another interesting study, Bryan et al evaluated the ability of glutathione to diminish the ischemia-reperfusion response in a canine model of lung autotransplantation.[97] They added reduced glutathione to the EC preservation solution and noted improved preservation as assessed by acute lung function and lung edema formation. The proposed mechanism relates to limitation of lipid peroxidation, as glutathione is oxidized by the enzyme glutathione peroxidase to reduce hydrogen peroxides and lipid peroxides to less toxic compounds.

As can be seen, considerable research is ongoing in the area of oxidant-induced lung injury. Clearly, with increasing knowledge in this field, further therapeutic manipulations will evolve to limit the ischemia induced reperfusion injury.

LUNG PRESERVATION TECHNIQUES

As noted in other sections, most currently used techniques for lung preservation involve hypothermic pulmonary artery flush. The technique employed by the Toronto Lung Transplant Program consists of an initial infusion of 1000 micrograms of PGE$_1$ into the pulmonary artery followed by a high volume (50ml/kg), low pressure pulmonary artery flush with modified EC. The tip of the left atrial appendage is excised to allow drainage of the flush solution. The lungs are ventilated with 100% oxygen throughout and then are hyperinflated to ensure there are no areas of atelectasis and then the trachea is clamped.[98]

At the University of Pittsburgh, the preservation technique is quite similar to that of the Toronto group, relying on PGE$_1$ pulmonary artery vasodilation followed by cold (4°C) EC flush. In a recent publication describing their technique no mention was made of lung hyperinflation, so whether this is important in their harvest method is unclear.[17]

Techniques for lobar harvest in living related donors require dissection and division of the donor vasculature prior to any flush. This obligates the graft to a period of normothermic ischemia prior to preservation. To remove the lobe in such a situation, the fissures are completed with a stapling device and then the donor is heparinized. The vasculature structures are divided followed by the bronchus. The reduced-size graft can then be flushed ex vivo to provide cooling. Clearly, this situation makes it difficult to administer pulmonary vasodilators prior to flush, although presumably they could be added to the flush solution. In addition, it is extremely difficult to remove a lobe from a hyperinflated lung, making it nearly impossible to avoid some degree of atelectasis in the donated lobe. Because of these factors, one might expect that acceptable lengths of ischemia in a living related donation would be considerably shorter.[11,99]

SUMMARY

Considerable progress has been made in the field of lung preservation over the past decade and acceptable graft function can now

be expected after ischemic times ranging up to 8 hours. Hypothermic flush, hyperinflation and prostaglandin pulmonary artery flushing are the cornerstones of the majority of clinically applied preservation techniques. Still, there is a considerable body of evidence available to suggest that further manipulations including limiting oxidant-induced lung injury will result in even longer acceptable ischemic intervals. In preserving the reduced-size pulmonary allograft, all of the above mentioned considerations apply regarding the relative intolerance of the lung to normothermic ischemia. Principals of preservation applicable to whole lung grafts are also appropriate in these reduced-size grafts, although techniques will have to be modified due to the constraints imposed by dissection and harvest of the pulmonary lobe.

REFERENCES

1. Reitz BA, Wallwork JL, Hunt SA et al. Heart-lung transplantation: successful therapy for patients with pulmonary vascular disease. N Eng J Med 1982; 306:557-64.
2. Toronto Lung Transplant Group. Unilateral lung transplantation for pulmonary fibrosis. N Engl J Med 1986; 314:1140-5.
3. Cooper JD. The evolution of techniques and indications for lung transplantation. Ann Surg 1990; 212:249-56.
4. Pasque MK, Cooper JD, Daiser LR et al. Improved technique for bilateral lung transplantation: rationale and initial clinical experience. Ann Thorac Surg 1990; 49:785-91.
5. Spray TL, Mallory GB, Conte CE, Huddleston CB, Kaiser LR. Pediatric lung transplantation for pulmonary hypertension and congenital heart disease. Ann Thorac Surg 1992; 54:216-25.
6. Starnes VA, Marshall SE, Leviston NJ et al. Heart-lung transplantation in infants, children and adolescents. J Pediatric Surg 1991; 26:434-38.
7. Starnes VA, Oyer PE, Bernstein D et al. Heart, heart-lung, and lung transplantation in the first year of life. Ann Thorac Surg 1992; 53:306-10.

8. Kaye MP. The Registry of the International Society for Heart and Lung Transplantation: The Official Report-1992. J Heart Lung Transplant 1992; 11:599-606.

9. Starnes V, Stoehr C, Theodor J, Lewiston N. Deciding to perform a living-donor lung transplantation: the paradigm. Poster presented at American Thoracic Society, Anaheim, CA, May 1991.

10. Kern JA, Tribble CG, Flanagan TL et al. Growth potential of porcine reduced-size mature pulmonary lobar transplants. J Thorac Cardiovasc Surg 1992; 104:1329-32.

11. Starnes VA, Lewiston NJ, Luikarb H et al. Current trends in lung transplantation. Lobar transplantation and expanded use of single lungs. J Thorac Cardiovasc Surg 1992; 104:1060-6.

12. Backer CL, Ohtake S, Zales VR et al. Living related lobar lung transplantation in beagle puppies. J Pediatric Surg 1991; 26:429-33.

13. Goldsmith MF. Mother to child: first living donor lung transplant. JAMA 1990; 264:2724.

14. Baldwin JC, Frist WH, Starkey TD et al. Distant graft procurable for combined heart and lung transplantation using pulmonary artery flush and simple topical hypothermia for graft preservation. Ann Thorac Surg 1987; 43:670-3.

15. Haydock DA, Low DE, Trulock ED et al. Pulmonary "twinning" procedure: use of lungs from one donor for single-lung transplantable in vivo recipients. Ann Thorac Surg 1992; 54:1189-92.

16. Todd TR, Goldberg M, Kosmal A et al. Separate extraction of cardiac and pulmonary graft from a single organ donor. Ann Thorac Surg 1988; 46:356-9.

17. Zenati M, Dowling RD, Armitage JM et al. Organ procurement for pulmonary transplantation. Ann Thorac Surg 1989; 48:882-6.

18. Haverich A, Scott WC, Jamieson SW et al. Twenty years of lung preservation - A review. J Heart Transplant 1985; 2:234-9.

19. Egan TM. Lung preservation. Seminars in thoracic and cardiovascular surgery 1992; 4:83-9.

20. Allison RC, Kyle J, Adkins WK et al. Effect of ischemia reperfusion or hypoxia reoxygenation on lung vascular permeability and resistance. J Appl Physiol 1990; 69:597-603.

21. Baumgartner WA, Reitz BA, Achuff SC (eds). Heart and Heart-Lung Transplantation WB Saunders, 1990; 319-71.

22. Toledo-Pereyra LH, Han T, Simmons RL et al. Lung preservation techniques. Ann Thorac Surg 1971; 23:487.

23. Siegelman SS, Sinha SBP, Veith FJ. Pulmonary reimplantation response. Ann Surg 1973; 177:30.

24. Blades B, Beattie EJ Jr, Hill RP et al. Ischemia of the lung. Ann Surg 1952; 136:56-62.

25. Egan TM, Lambert CJ, Reddick R. A strategy to increase the donor pool: The use of cadaver lungs for transplantation. Ann Thorac Surg 1991; 52:1113-21.

26. Stevens GH, Sanchez MM, Chappell GL. Enhancement of lung preservation by prevention of lung collapse. J Surg Res 1973; 14:400-05.

27. Fonkalsrud EW, Sanchez MM, Lassaletta L et al. Extended preservation of the ischemic canine lung by ventilation with PEEP. J Surg Res 1975; 18:437-45.

28. Puskas JD, Hitai T, Christie N et al. Reliable thirty-hour lung preservation by donor lung hyperinflation. J Thorac Cardiovasc Surg 1992; 104:1075-82.

29. Fisher AB, Dodia C, Tan Z, Ayene I, Eckenoff RC. Oxygen-dependent lipid peroxidation during lung ischemia. J Clin Invest 1991; 88:674-79.

30. Allison RC Kyle J, Adkins WK et al. Effect of ischemia-reperfusion or hypoxia-reoxygenation on lung vascular permeability and resistance. J Appl Physiol 1990; 69:597-603.

31. Granger PN. Role of xanthine oxidase and granulocytes in ischemia-reperfusion injury. Am J Physiol 1988; 255:H1269-H1275.

32. Kennedy TP, Rao NN, Hopkins C et al. Role of reactive oxygen species in reperfusion injury of the rabbit lung. J Clin Invest 1985; 83:1326-35.

33. Fridovich I. The history of oxygen radicals. Science 1978; 201:875.

34. White BC, Kravse GS, Aust SD, Eyster GE. Post ischemic tissue injury by iron mediated free radical lipid peroxidation. Ann Emerg Med 1985; 14:804.

35. Gutteridge JMC, Richmond R, Halliwell B. Inhibitor of iron catalyzed formation of hydroxyl radicals from superoxide and of lipid peroxidal by deferoxamine. Biochem J 1979; 184:469.

36. Schanne FAX, Kane AB, Young EE, Farber JL. Calcium dependence of toxic cell death: a final common pathway. Science 1979; 206:700.

37. Leter AM. Eicosonoilds as mediators of ischemia and shock. Fed Proc 1985; 44:275.

38. Adkins WK, Taylor AE. Role of xanthine oxidase and neutrophils in ischemia-reperfusion injury in rabbit lung. J Appl Physiol 1990; 69:2012-18.

39. Klavsner JM, Paterson IS, Goldman G et al. Postischemic renal injury is mediated by neutrophils and leukotrines. Am J Physiol 1989; 256:F794-F802.

40. Sewall H. Henry Newell Martin: Professor of Biology in Johns Hopkins University, 1876-1893. Johns Hopkins Hospital Bulletin 1911; 22:327.

41. Knowlton FP, Starling EH. The influence of variations in temperature and blood-pressure on the performance of the isolated mammalian heart. J Physiol 1912-13; 44:206.

42. Robicsek F, Sawyer PW, Taylor FH. Simple method of keeping the heart "alive" and functioning outside the body for prolong periods. Surgery 1963; 53:525.

43. Hardesty RL, Griffith BP, Autoperfusion of the heart and lungs for preservation during distant procurement. J Thorac Cardiovasc Surg 1987; 93:11.

44. Reitz, BA. Personal communication.

45. Wang LS, Yoshikawa K, Miyoshi S et al. The effect of ischemic time and temperature on lung preservation in a simple ex vivo rabbit model used for functional assessment. J Thorac Cardiovasc Surg 1989; 98:333-42.

46. Fraser CD, Tamura F, Adachi H et al. Donor core-cooling provides improved static preservation for heart-lung transplantation.

Ann Thorac Surg 1988; 45:253-7.

47. Pillai R, Fraser CD, Bando K et al. Core-cooling remains the most effective technique of extended heart-lung preservation: further experimental evidence. Transplant Proc 1990; 22:551-552.

48. Baumgartner WA, Williams GM, Fraser CD. Cardiopulmonary bypass with profound hypothermia: an optimal preservation method for multiorgan preservation. Transplantation 1987; 47:124-127.

49. Fujimura S, Handa M, Kondo T et al. Successful 48-hour simple hypothermic preservation of canine lung transplants. Transplant Proc 1987; 19:1334-6.

50. Liang-Shun W, Nakamoto K, Chia-Mong H, Shinichird M, Cooper JD. Influence of temperature of flushing solution on lung preservation. Ann Thorac Surg 1993; 55:771-5.

51. Otto G, Wolff H, Jerlings I, Gellert K. Preservation damage in liver transplantation: influence of rapid cooling. Transplantation 1985; 42:122-4.

52. Swearson KD, Dufek JH, Kahn DR. Improved myocardial preservation at 4°C. Ann Thorac Surg 31980; 0:519-26.

53. Wahlers T, Haverich A, Fieguth HG et al. Flush perfusion using Euro-Collins solution vs cooling by means of extracorporeal circulation in heart-lung preservation. J Heart Transplant 1986; 5:89-98.

54. Keenan RJ, Griffith BP, Kormos RL, Armitage JM, Hardesty RL. Increased perioperative lung preservation injury with lung procurement by Euro-Collins solution flush. J Heart Lung Transplant 1991; 10:650-5.

55. Wahlberg JA, Love R, Landegaard L, Southard JH, Belzer FO. 72 hour preservation of the pancreas. Transplantation 1986; 43:5-8.

56. Henry ML, Somma BG, Ferguson RM. Improved immediate function of renal allografts with Belzer perfusate. Transplantation 198845:73-5; .

57. Todo S, Nery J, Yanaga K, Poderta L, Gordon RD, Starzl TS. Extended preservation of human liver grafts with UW solution. JAMA 1989; 261:711-4.

58. Unruh HW. Vascular and interstitial effect of University of Wisconsin solution in canine lung. Ann Thorac Surg 1992; 54:1168-71.

59. Semik M, Moller F, Bernhard A, Toomes H. Comparison of Euro-Collins and UW solutions for lung preservation using the parabiotic rat perfusion model. Transplant Proc 1990; 22:2235-36.

60. Hirt SW, Wahlers T, Jurmann MJ et al. University of Wisconsin versus modified Euro-Collins solution for lung preservation. Ann Thorac Surg 1992; 53:74-9.

61. Naka Y, Shirakura R, Matsuda H et al. Canine heart-lung transplantation after twenty-four hour hypothermic preservation. J Heart Lung Transplant 1991; 10:296-303.

62. Hardesty RL, Aeba R, Armitage JM, Kormos RL, Griffith BP. A clinical trial of University of Wisconsin solution for pulmonary preservation. J Thorac Cardiovasc Surg 1993; 105:660-6.

63. Steen S, Sjoberg T, Massa G, Ericsson L, Lindberg L. Safe pulmonary preservation for 12 hours with low potassium-dextran solution. Ann Thorac Surg 1993; 55:434-40.

64. Pvskas JD, Cardoso PF, Mayer E et al. Equivalent eighteen-hour lung preservation with low potassium dextran or Euro-Collins solution after prostaglandin E1 infusion. J Thorac Cardiovasc Surg 1992; 104:83-9.

65. Yamaraki F, Yokomise H, Keshavjeg SH et al. The superiority of an extracellular fluid solution over Euro-Collins solution for pulmonary preservation. Transplantation 1990; 49:690-4.

66. Hooper TL, Locke TS, Fetherston G, Flecknell PA, McGregor CG. Comparison of cold flush perfusion with modified blood versus modified Euro-Collins solution for lung preservation. J Heart Transplant 1990; 9:429-34.

67. Kadowitz PJ, Chapnick BM, Feigin LP et al. Pulmonary and systemic vasodilation effects of the newly discovered prostaglandin PGI2. J Appl Physiol 1978; 45:408-13.

68. Yamashita C, Dobo H, Fukumasa T et al. Effect of prostaglandin I2 and superoxide dismutase on reperfusion injury of warm ischemic lung. Ann Thorac Surg 1992; 54:921-4.

69. Leter AM, Ogletree ML, Smith JB et al. Prostacyclin: a potentially valuable agent for preserving myocardial tissue in acute myocardial ischemia. Science 1978; 200:52.

70. Jones G, Hurley JV. The effect of prostacyclin in the adhesion of leukocytes to injured vascular endothelium. J Pathol 1984; 142:51-9.

71. Baldwin JC, Harjula A, Starkey TD, Jamieson SW, Shumway NE. Improved heart-lung graft preservation with prostaglandin E1. J Am Coll Cardiol 1987; 9:29A.

72. Harjula AJ, Baldwin JC. Lung transplantation in the pig with successful preservation using prostaglandin E1. J Appl Cardiol 1987; 2:397-402.

73. Bonser RS, Fragomeni LS, Jamieson SW et al. The use of PGE1 in 12 hour lung preservation. J Heart Transplant 1990; 9:70.

74. Bonser RS, Fracomen LS, Jamieson SW, Kaye MP. Deleterious affects of prostaglandin E1 in 12 hour lung preservation. Br Heart J 1989; 61:463.

75. Veno T, Yokomise H, Oka T et al. The effect of PGE1 and temperature on lung function following preservation. Transplantation 1991; 52:626-30.

76. Novick RJ, Reid KR, Denning L et al. Prolonged preservation of canine lung allografts: the role of prostaglandins. Ann Thorac Surg 1991; 51:853.

77. Golub M, Zia P, Matsuno M, Horton R. Metabolism of prostaglandin A1 and E1 in man. J Clin Invest 1975; 56:1404-10.

78. Moncada S, Gryglewski R, Bunting S, Vane JR. An enzyme isolated from arteries transforms prostaglandin endoperoxides to an unstable substance that inhibits platelet aggregation. Nature 1976; 263:663-5.

79. Mulvin D, Jones K, Howard R, Grosso M, Repine J. The effect of prostacyclin as a constintuent of a preservation solution in protecting lungs from ischemic injury because of its vasodilator properties. Transplantation 1990; 49:828-30.

80. Hooper TL, Thomson DS, Jones MT et al. Amelioration of lung ischemic injury with

prostacyclin. Transplantation 1990; 49:1031-35.

81. Inui K, Schafer HJ, Aoki M et al. Effect of methylprednisolone and prostaglandin on bronchial perfusion in lung transplantation. Ann Thorac Surg 1993; 55:464-9.

82. Klepetko W, Louninger A, Wisser W et al. Pulmonary surfactant in bronchoalveolar lavage after canine lung transplantation: effect of L-carnitine application. J Thorac Cardiovasc Surg 1990; 99:1048-58.

83. Suzuki M, Inaven W, Kvietys M et al. Superoxide mediates reperfusion-induced leukocyte endothelial cell interactions. Am J Physiol 1989; 257:H1740-45.

84. Breda MA, Hall TS, Stuart RS et al. Twenty-four hour lung preservation by hypothermia and leukocyte depletion. J heart Transplant 1985; 4:325-9.

85. Schueler S, DeValeria P, Hatanaka M et al. Successful 24-hour lung preservation with donor core-cooling and leukocyte depletion in an orthotopic double-lung transplant model. J Thorac Cardiovasc Surg 1992; 104:273-82.

86. Pillai R, Bando K, Schueler S et al. Leukocyte depletion results in excellent heart-lung function after 12 hours of storage. Ann Thorac Surg 1990; 50:271-4l.

87. Alba M, Yokoyama Y, Snow R et al. Effects of allopurinol pretreatment with pulmonary flush on lung preservation. J Heart Lung Transplant 1992; 11:1025-30.

88. Qayumi AK, Jamieson WR, Godin DW et al. Response to allopurinol pretreatment in a swine model of heart-lung transplantation. J Invest Surg 1990; 3:331-40.

89. Bonser RS, Fragomeni LS, Edwards BJ et al. Allopurinol and deferroxamine improve canine lung preservation. Transplant Proc 1990; 22:557-8.

90. Stuart RS, Baumgartner WA, Borkon AM et al. Five-hour hypothermic lung preservation with oxygen free-radical scavengers.

Transplant Proc 1985; 17:1454-6.

91. Pickford MA, Gower JD, Dore C, Fryer PR, Green CJ. Lipid peroxidation and ultrastructural changes in rate lung isografts after single-passage organ flush and 48-hour cold storage with and without one-hour reperfusion in vivo. Transplantation 1990; 50:210-18.

92. Braugher JM, Pregenzer JF, Chase RL et al. Novel 21 amino-steroids as potent inhibitors of iron-dependent lipid peroxidation. J Biol Chem 1987; 262:10438-40.

93. Aeba R, Killinger W, Keenan R et al. Lazaroid U74500A as an additive to the University of Wisconsin solution for pulmonary grafts in the rat transplant model. J Thorac Cardiovasc Surg 1992; 104:1333-9.

94. Holzgrete HH, Buchanan LV, Gibson JK. Effect of U74006F, a novel inhibitor of lipid peroxidation in stunned reperfused canine myocardium. J Cardiovasc Pharm 1990; 15:239-48.

95. Vercelloti GM, Huh PW, Yin HQ et al. Enhancement of PMN mediated endothelial damage by PAF; PAF primes PMN responses to activating stimuli. Clin Res 1986; 34:917-22.

96. Corcoran PC, Wang Y, Katz NM et al. Platelet activating factor antagonist enhances lung preservation in a canine model of single lung allotransplantation. J Thorac Cardiovasc Surg 1992; 104:66-72.

97. Bryan CL, Cohen DJ, Dew JA, Trinkle JK, Jenkinson SG. Glutathione decreases the pulmonary reimplantation response in canine lung autotransplants. Chest 1991; 100:1694-702.

98. Christie NA, Waddell TK. Lung preservation. Chest Surg Clin North Am 1993; 3:29-47.

99. Crombleholme TM, Adzick NS, Longaker MT et al. Reduced-size lung transplantation in neonatal swine: technique and short-term physiologic response. Ann Thorac Surg 1990; 49:55-60.

CHAPTER 4

EXPERIMENTAL REDUCED-SIZE LUNG TRANSPLANTATION: MODELS, EXPERIMENTAL TECHNIQUES AND METHODS, PITFALLS

Scott E. Langenburg
Curtis G. Tribble

INTRODUCTION

Experimental lung transplantation in animals is crucial to our understanding of postoperative growth and function of human lung transplants. Without experimentation, pioneers in reduced-size lung transplantation would lack direction and the basic understanding of techniques and postoperative changes in pulmonary function to adequately care for patients. Because clinical reduced-size lung transplantation has yet to result in long-term success, data of long-term function of these specialized grafts need to be gathered from studies performed in experimental models.

Reduced-size Lung Transplantation, edited by John A. Kern, M.D. and Irving L. Kron, M.D.; © 1993 R.G. Landes Company.

Over the past four decades several animal models have been used for experimental lung transplantation including porcine, canine, primate, rat and ovine. Canine models were the first to be used to explore the consequences of lung transplantation. The first reported pulmonary allograft was by H. Metras in 1950 using a canine model.[1] The dog model was also used by many other early researchers, however, early canine lung transplantation was plagued by frequent postoperative death from infection and rejection.[2,3] As a result, other animal models have been developed. Primate models have been used to evaluate allograft pathology, allograft physiology and the effect of denervation on respiratory function[4-6] and a rat model has been utilized to evaluate rejection in lung allografts and growth of immature lung allografts.[7-9]

REDUCED-SIZE LUNG TRANSPLANTATION

The choice of transplant model for studying reduced-size lung allografts can be based on what species the investigator is most familiar with. In the thoracic and cardiovascular research laboratory at the University of Virginia we have chosen to use a porcine model. This decision is based on our familiarity with this animal and the fact that neonatal swine pulmonary architecture and development parallels that of humans.[10] Other research groups have also chosen this model, while some investigators with documented models of reduced-size lung transplantation have utilized dogs and lambs.[11-17] The porcine model has demonstrated that pigs have the ability to withstand thoracotomy and lung transplantation with acceptable operative mortality (10–20%) and this mortality is generally lower than in most other reported models of experimental lung transplantation. Specifically, this ability to withstand a major operation can be lacking in canine models.

Crombleholme was probably the first to describe the technique of experimental reduced-size lung transplantation and also used a porcine model.[11,12] Wain and his colleagues from Boston have utilized in an ovine model, the right upper lobe from an adult donor (which

allows better size match), heterotopically transplanted into the left chest cavity of a neonatal recipient.[15,16] Backer and his colleagues from Chicago developed a chronic canine model of reduced-size lung transplantation which involved orthotopic transplantation of a mature left lower lobe into a living-related puppy.[14] Finally, Lillehei, Everts and Shamberger, also from Boston, have reported long-term survival in neonatal lambs after either heterotopic or orthotopic transplantation of reduced-size mature lobes from adult sheep.[17] It appears that several viable animal models of reduced-size lung transplantation are presently available.

OPERATIVE TECHNIQUE AND EXPERIMENTAL METHODOLOGY

In this section the technical aspects of porcine reduced-size lung transplantation will be described as performed at the University of Virginia. Comments will be made on other models and approaches as they have been reported in the literature. We will also outline experimental techniques which we have used to evaluate the transplanted lungs postoperatively as a guide for other investigators who may be interested in this area.

OPERATIVE TECHNIQUE

Preoperative preparation

Eight to ten-week-old piglets are prepared as recipients for the reduced-size mature lobar transplant by receiving aspirin for two consecutive days preoperatively. Use of aspirin has decreased the incidence of pulmonary vein thrombosis which plagued our earlier attempts of experimental lung transplantation. The piglets are also given cyclosporine (18 mg/kg, PO) the day prior to the operation and preoperative antibiotics (ampicillin 250 mg, IV, bid and chloramphenicol 250 mg, IV, bid). We have found that using piglets younger than eight weeks makes the procedure technically more difficult and the smaller animals are not as able to withstand the operation.

Anesthesia

The animals are sedated with intramuscular ketamine (10 mg/kg) and are intubated and placed on a volume ventilator at 10-20 cc/kg and a rate of 12-15 breaths per minute. A 20 gauge angiocatheter is placed in an ear vein to administer fluid, antibiotics, heparin, and immunosuppressive agents. End-tidal CO_2 is used to monitor adequacy of ventilation and adjust respiratory rate and tidal volume. Supplemental oxygen is provided to achieve an arterial blood oxygen tension (PaO_2) of greater than 100 mmHg. Anesthesia is maintained using halothane (0.5–1.5%). Care must be taken to not use more halothane than necessary for adequate anesthesia because of halothane cardiac toxicity and intraoperative death. Intravenous pentobarbital is utilized to supplement the halothane as needed (5 mg IV push). Paralytics are seldom needed in the smaller animals (recipients). However, dissection in larger animals (donors) is sometimes facilitated by their use (metocurine 100 mg/kg, IV push). Continuous arterial blood pressure monitoring is not necessary.

General operative techniques

Our laboratory utilizes a model for reduced-size pulmonary lobar transplantation that involves using a fully mature left lower lobe transplanted orthotopically into an immature animal. Donors and recipients are obtained from the same supplier and are generally of the same brood. Blood and tissue typing are not routinely done. (It is important, however, to obtain healthy animals free of disease.) Donor lobes are harvested from sexually mature pigs of either sex. The donor pigs are at least six months old and usually weigh in excess of 100 kg. Previous studies by other researchers of pulmonary development have shown that most aspects of postnatal porcine lung development are complete by three months.[10] The use of donor pigs older than three months assures that the transplanted reduced-size lobe is fully mature at the time of transplantation into the young piglet. Our studies have shown that although the donor mature left lower lobe is approximately three times the size of the explanted recipient's

entire immature left lung, transplantation can be successfully accomplished. In cases of extreme size mismatch, the donor lobe can be sculpted to fit the recipient chest cavity using a surgical stapler as described by Crombleholme.[12]

Donor operation

After intubation and adequate anesthesia the adult donor is placed in a right side down position. The skin is sterilized with iodine scrub, 70% isopropyl alcohol, and iodine prep solution and then sterilely draped. A left posterolateral thoracotomy is performed over the fifth intercostal space and carried down through the muscle layers with electrocautery. After placement of a rib spreader, the left upper lobe is reflected to expose the hemiazygous vein. This is ligated and divided to allow better exposure of the left pulmonary artery. The pulmonary artery, superior pulmonary vein and bronchus are then isolated and encircled by silastic vessel loops. The inferior pulmonary ligament is sharply divided and the lower lobe reflected cephalad. The inferior pulmonary vein is isolated and also encircled by a vessel loop. Before clamping the vessels and left mainstem bronchus, heparin is given (100 U/kg, IV) and allowed to circulate for five minutes. The pulmonary artery, pulmonary veins and bronchus, respectively, are then clamped and divided. Care is taken to take as much of the vessels and bronchus with the specimen so that they can be fine tuned to fit the recipient's anatomy. It has been our practice to then euthanize the donor animal with a lethal injection of pentobarbital. Other groups have reported that the hilar structures can be oversewn and the chest closed, thus preserving the life of the donor.[11,12,14–16]

Lung preparation

Once removed from the donor, the lung is immersed in sterile ice-cold heparinized saline slush and the pulmonary artery is gently and slowly perfused with cold heparinized physiologic saline until the effluent from the pulmonary veins is clear. The upper lobe is removed and the vessels and bronchus are trimmed to appropriate sizes. Other groups have described, and we have also utilized, the technique of in vivo dissection of the lobe to be transplanted. We have found that in vivo dissection can shorten the cold ischemic time of the transplanted lobe.

Recipient operation

As the mature lobe is being recovered from the donor the recipient piglet is prepared for transplantation in a similar fashion as described for the donor. Dissection is performed in an identical fashion. The recipient is prepared by the time the donor lobe is ready in order to minimize ischemic time. Two operating teams facilitate the process. It should be noted that once the left mainstem bronchus of the recipient piglet is clamped the tidal volume should be decreased to minimize the risk of barotrauma to the contralateral lung.

Reduced-size lobar transplant

Once the recipient animal and donor lobe are prepared, the reduced-size graft is appropriately positioned in the left chest and the inferior pulmonary vein is approximated end-to-end with a running 7-0 monofilament polyglyconate suture (Maxon, Davis-Geck), (Fig. 1). Other investigators have described the technique of anastomosing the donor vein, with a patch of atrium, directly to the left atrial appendage of the recipient so as to avoid placing a clamp on the left atrium and impairing venous return.[11,12] (Fig. 1) This is a technique which we have also used in some instances. The bronchus is then approximated using a telescoping (size mismatch) or end-to-end anastomosis with 4-0

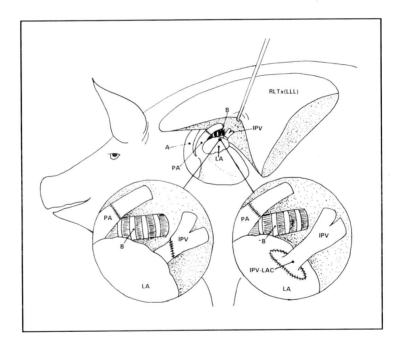

Fig. 1. Diagrammatic representation of porcine reduced-size lung transplant using an allograft left lower lobe. The venous anastomosis can be done in a spatulated end-to-end technique (left inset) or by harvesting a patch of left atrium around the donor vein which is then sewn to the left atrial appendage of the recipient (right inset) as described by Crombleholme.(11,12)
A=aorta, B=bronchus, PA=pulmonary artery, IPV=inferior pulmonary vein, LA=left atrium, RLTx-LLL=reduced-size lobar transplant-left lower lobe, IPV-LAC=inferior pulmonary vein-left atrial cuff.

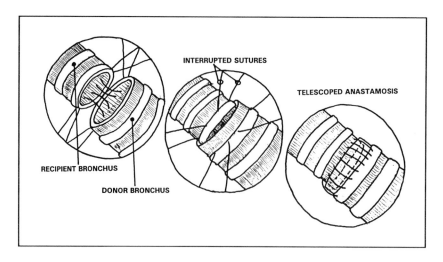

Fig. 2. Bronchial anastomosis of porcine left lower lobe reduced-size lung transplant using a mild telescoping technique.

monofilament polyglyconate interrupted simple stitches (Fig. 2). The bronchial clamp is removed and several tidal volumes are delivered without allowing the expiratory phase to occur (stacking the inspirations). Stacking re-expands the lobe and tests the anastomosis for air leaks, which if present and small are usually well tolerated and close spontaneously. Omentopexy has been found to be unnecessary in our porcine model as long as excessive dissection of the recipient bronchus is avoided and the donor bronchus is not too long. The pulmonary artery is then approximated using a running 6-0 monofilament polyglyconate suture. At this point another dose of intravenous heparin is given (100 U/kg) to assure proper anticoagulation and prevent of pulmonary venous and arterial thrombosis. Before the suture on the pulmonary artery is secured, the pulmonary veins are allowed to back bleed and rid the pulmonary circulation of air. The arterial suture is then secured and the arterial clamp is removed. All anastomoses are examined for hemostasis. A tube thoracostomy is then performed and the wound is closed. The tube is placed on suction using a three chamber system. Lung ischemic times generally range from 90 to 160 minutes.

Postoperative care

At the completion of the procedure the animals are allowed to awaken under close supervision. Once breathing well spontaneously, usually 15-30 minutes after stopping the anesthetics, the pigs are extubated. The tube thoracostomy is removed 24 hours postoperatively while the animal receives inhaled halothane. Warming lights are provided in the early postoperative period.

As mentioned earlier, the animals receive two preoperative days of aspirin (325 mg, PO). Aspirin is continued postoperatively every day for seven days, then every other day until the animals are euthanized after final studies. The animals receive postoperative antibiotics (ampicillin 250 mg, IV, bid and chloramphenicol 250 mg, IV, bid) for four days. The immunosuppressive regimen consists of: 1) cyclosporine (18 mg/kg, PO QD) starting one day preoperatively and continuing for the life of the animal, 2) azathioprine (1 mg/kg, PO QD) given during the operation (IV) and every day for the life of the animal, 3) methylprednisolone (500 mg, IV bid) starting on the day of operation and continuing for four days. Long-term steroids are not routinely administered. Chest roentgenograms are performed at one week and then monthly for the life of the animal (Fig. 3). Diagnosis of rejection is made on the basis of increased temperature, lethargy, tachypnea, anorexia or coughing. Animals thought to be rejecting do not routinely have chest roentgenography performed because of the hazard of sedation in a compromised animal. Treatment consists of empiric pulse steroids (methylprednisolone 500 mg, IM bid) and antibiotics (ampicillin 250 mg, IV bid and chloramphenicol 250 mg IV bid) for four days.

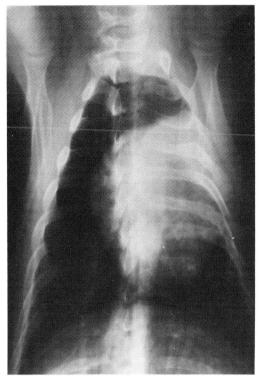

A

Fig. 3. Chest radiographs of reduced-size porcine lung transplants taken (A) 10 days after transplant and (B) 3 months after transplant. A chest radiograph of a normal pig is also shown (C) for the sake of comparison.

C

B

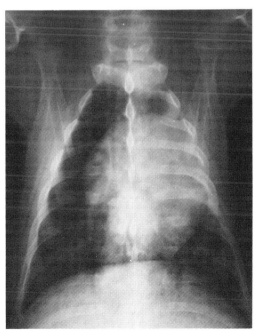

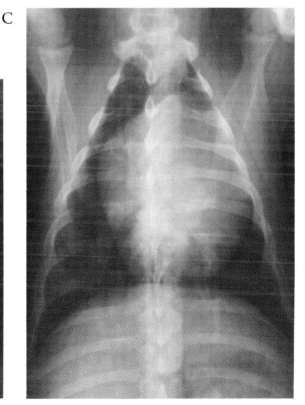

Experimental study methods

Animals are allowed to grow for a specified time, following which the reduced-size transplants are studied functionally and morphometrically. During the period of growth, which in our studies has been 10 weeks to three months, the young pigs usually increase their weight approximately 300-400%. We have evaluated several parameters of lung function and growth including pulmonary mechanics and functional lung volumes, gas exchange, pulmonary hemodynamics, vascular endothelial function, lung morphology, extravascular lung water and vascular smooth muscle content. The experimental techniques used in these evaluations will be described below. These protocols can be carried out at any point during the postoperative course. However, most are terminal studies and the animals are generally euthanized following the study.

Pulmonary mechanics and gas exchange

Animals are sedated and anesthetized using ketamine, pentobarbital and metocurine, and a tracheotomy is made. The animals are ventilated at 10–15 ml/kg and a respiratory rate adequate to maintain normal pCO_2. Halothane is avoided at this time because of its effects on pulmonary physiology. A six centimeter latex balloon (2 ml volume, inflated) is passed into the lower third of the esophagus and is used for measurement of transpulmonary pressure. Air flow is measured at the airway (trachea) opening with a pneumotachometer connected to a differential transducer attached through an analog to digital converter to a microcomputer. Prior to study the pneumotachometer should be calibrated with a standard gas rotameter and all calibrations recorded on the microcomputer. Transrespiratory pressure (the difference between airway and esophageal pressures) is measured with a transducer which is also attached to the microcomputer. Pressure volume loops are created for several breaths at different tidal volumes and respiratory rates from which calculations of dynamic and static compliance and dynamic resistance can be obtained. Dynamic compliance is calculated

as the slope of the line of best fit through the origin and apex of the pressure-volume loop. Dynamic resistance is calculated from measurements of the total (inspiratory and expiratory) pressure change at 50% tidal volume divided by the absolute value of flow at this volume. Static compliance is calculated by dividing the inflation volume (200, 400, 600 ml, etc.) by the corresponding airway pressure at that volume. These measurements are corrected for functional residual capacity by dividing the above result by the calculated functional residual capacity.

Functional residual capacity (FRC) is measured using the helium-dilution method. The pig is ventilated, beginning at end-expiration, through the endotracheal tube connector with a calibrated syringe containing a known concentration of helium mixed with sufficient oxygen to maintain baseline FIO_2. The inflation volume is equal to the tidal volume, adjusted for the experimental conditions. The pigs are ventilated with this gas mixture until the helium concentration reaches equilibrium, usually in 1–2 minutes. The final volume of gas and helium in the syringe is measured and the FRC is calculated with Boyle's equation: $FRC=((C1*V1)/C2)-V1$; where $C1$=initial helium concentration; $C2$=final concentration of helium; $V1$=initial volume. The studies described above can be done serially by allowing the animals to recover between measurements.

Function of the reduced-size transplant is evaluated by isolating the allograft in vivo. Isolation of the left sided graft is accomplished by passing balloon catheters into the right main stem and epi-arterial bronchi. Catheters are positioned bronchoscopically. With these occlusive catheters in place selective ventilation of the lobar allograft can be done allowing measurements of air flow, pulmonary mechanics and FRC as described above. Similar studies can be made of the right lung after occlusion of the left mainstem bronchus.

Pulmonary hemodynamics

At the time of transplantation baseline hemodynamic measurements can be obtained.

Pulmonary artery catheters are utilized to obtain pulmonary artery pressure, pulmonary capillary wedge pressure and cardiac output by the thermal-dilution technique. Alternatively, other investigators have evaluated graft hemodynamics acutely with ultrasonic flow probes placed around the allograft left lower lobe (LLL FLOW) and main pulmonary arteries.[11,12,15] Pressure measurements of the left atrium (LAP) and pulmonary artery (PAP) are obtained using needles or indwelling catheters attached to transducers. Pulmonary vascular resistance (PVR) can be calculated for the transplanted lobe using the formula PVR=PAP-LAP/LLL FLOW. Terminal studies are done in our laboratory utilizing a median sternotomy so that both pulmonary arteries can be manipulated and the indwelling pulmonary artery catheter placed in the pulmonary artery to be studied. With both pulmonary arteries isolated right- and left-sided hemodynamic measurements can be obtained. Most importantly, contralateral cross-clamping of the pulmonary artery can allow evaluation of capillary recruitment of the allograft (or native right lung) in response to increased flow. Systemic blood gases can also be obtained at this time to assess gas exchange of the allograft or native right lung. Other manipulations, such as assessing the vascular response to hypoxemia can also be done in these acute experiments.

Pulmonary vascular endothelial function (endothelial dependent and independent relaxation)

Pulmonary artery endothelial function can be studied using two different techniques: vascular ring model and prostacyclin production.[18,19] The vascular ring model assesses endothelium-derived relaxing factor (EDRF) activity.[18] The model uses intraparenchymal pulmonary artery segments (internal diameter 3–4 mm) harvested from the transplanted lung and carefully cleaned connective tissue. The segments (3 mm wide) are suspended in a water-jacketed tissue bath containing Krebs-Henseleit buffer and connected to force

transducers for isometric tension measurements. Indomethacin ($10E-5$ M) is added to the baths to inhibit prostacyclin synthesis by blocking cyclooxygenase activity.[19] The rings are allowed to equilibrate for one hour at a resting tension predetermined by the generation of length tension curves to achieve 75% maximal tension prior to constriction with phenylephrine, an alpha-adrenergic agonist. Cumulative dose-dependent relaxation response curves are then determined to methacholine (a stable analogue of acetylcholine) to evaluate for endothelial-dependent relaxation and to sodium nitroprusside to test for endothelial-independent relaxation. Results are expressed as dose-dependent percent relaxation after phenylephrine contraction.

Prostacyclin, a potent vasodilator and inhibitor of platelet aggregation, is predominantly produced by vascular endothelium. It is a labile substance and spontaneously hydrolyzes to the stable but inactive 6-keto-prostaglandin-F-1-alpha. Prostacyclin production at both basal and stimulated states can be determined. Arachidonic acid, the precursor of prostacyclin, is used to stimulate prostacyclin synthesis. Assays can be performed in parallel with the vascular ring experiments from baths that are not exposed to indomethacin. Aliquots of buffer are removed from the baths before and after the addition of arachidonic acid. Radioimmunoassays for 6-keto-prostaglandin F 1-alpha can then be run to assess the picograms of immunoreactive product per milligram of wet weight of vascular ring.[19]

Lung morphometry

Following all functional studies of airway mechanics and pulmonary hemodynamics, the heart-lung blocks are removed after heparinization and euthanasia with a lethal injection of pentobarbital. The heart and lungs are separated and flushed with saline. An intraparenchymal arterial segment is obtained for vascular ring analysis and a few grams of parenchyma are obtained and frozen for subsequent evaluation of extravascular lung water to calculate dry lung weights. Wet weights of the lungs, left ventricle and septum, and right ventricular free wall are obtained. Anastomotic areas are measured. The lungs are fixed with buffered formalin (10%) instilled into the airway and artery at a constant pressure of 25 cm H_2O. After at least seven days of fixation, postfixation volume is measured by the water displacement method.[20] The lungs are then cut into one centimeter thick parallel slices extending from the hilum to the periphery. Morphometry is carried out at three levels using a technique proposed by Gil[21] based on the point-counting method of Dunnill.[22] The first level determines the parenchymal volume percent by point-counting the lung slices, with exclusion of all airways and vessels greater than one millimeter. The second level involves determinations of volume proportions of alveolar air spaces and alveolar duct air spaces using microscopic point-counting under low magnification. The third level determines volume density of the septa in the true parenchyma by differential point-counting under higher magnification. This level also includes examination of specific elements, such as: 1) capillaries, 2) cross-sectional surface area of the alveoli and airways by tracing the perimeters of 100 alveoli and 50 noncartilaginous airways on a video monitor with a manual cursor. Total alveolar number is determined by using the counting principle of Weibel and Gomez.[23] In addition to these parameters others have used digitized computed tomography and a nitrogen washout technique to evaluate lung volume.[24]

Extravascular lung water determination

Extravascular lung water measurement is begun by determining hemoglobin and vascular water content of the blood and by homogenizing lung tissue in an equal volume of distilled water. The homogenized lung tissue is then divided into two samples. The first is placed in a vacuum drying oven at 40°C, and the second is centrifuged to create a supernatant. The supernatant is further divided, one portion to be dried to determine water content and the second analyzed for hemoglobin content. Lung water is determined by the equations:

$$QB=Qh*(HgS/HgB)*(FWH/FWS)*(DB/DS); \quad Qwl=(QH*FWH)-(QB*FWB)-(Q+W);$$ and $$dQl=QH-QB-Qwl-(Q+B),$$ where QB=residual blood content, Qh=weight of homogenate, Hb=hemoglobin content of supernatant (S) or blood (B), FW=fractional water content of homogenate (H) of supernatant (S), Qwl=water mass of blood-free lung, Q+W=amount of water added to lung during homogenation, dQl=dry lung mass.[25,26]

Vascular smooth muscle content determination

Specimens of pulmonary arteries are stored in 10% formaldehyde at 4°C for 24 hours and then fixed in paraffin. Sections 3–4 µm thick are stained using the immunoperoxidase technique. The sections are then deparaffinized, hydrated and washed in phosphate-buffered saline (PBS) for five minutes. Quenching of endogenous peroxidase activity is accomplished by incubation of the specimens for thirty minutes in 0.3% H_2O_2 diluted in methanol. Sections are then washed for 20 minutes in PBS, incubated for 20 minutes with normal horse serum and then incubated for 90 minutes with the mouse B4 actin specific monoclonal antibody diluted 1:100 in PBS. They are rinsed in PBS and incubated with anti-murine IgG biotinylated antibody for 30 minutes. Sections are again washed in PBS (10 minutes) and incubated for 45 minutes in avidin-biotinylated horseradish peroxidase complex and then exposed to 0.1% diaminobenzidine tetrachloride and 0.02% for five minutes. Sections are finally washed in water and counterstained with hematoxylin. Differential cross-sectional areas of total capillary surface area and stained smooth muscle are determined with a microscopic analysis system. Measurements are expressed as a ratio of smooth muscle area to capillary surface area. These results are then correlated with measurements of pulmonary vascular compliance. Negative controls are done by having the primary antibody replaced by either the antibody preabsorbed with actin or by a nonimmune antibody (MOPC 21 protein), and staining is again assessed and quantified.[28]

PITFALLS

In the past, the canine model was not particularly conducive to long-term survival following experimental lung transplantation. The porcine model, however, has done very well. We now have approximately seven years experience with lobar transplantation in the pig. The operation is performed with approximately an 80–85% short-term survival and 70–75% long-term survival. Although the porcine model is an excellent one, the ultimate question remains: does this animal model correlate with clinical pediatric reduced-size lung transplantation?

In addition to the problem of extrapolating animal data to clinical situations the technical aspects of animal lung transplantation can present several challenges. The technique is not simple and requires a great deal of time to learn and perfect. Operative expertise plays an important role in the success of experimental lung transplantation. Technical errors can result in failure of any of the anastomoses, vascular or bronchial, due to stricture or leak. In addition, anastomotic problems can occur even despite excellent technique. Pulmonary venous thrombosis is particularly troublesome. We attempt to prevent pulmonary venous thrombosis with systemic heparinization prior to initial cross-clamping and again just prior to removing the clamps, and by the administration of aspirin several days prior to transplantation and daily postoperatively.

Postoperative care of the animals can also be challenging. As with an immunosuppressed host the risk of infection is an ever present problem. In porcine lung transplant recipients the diagnosis of infection is made more difficult because symptoms of rejection and infection are very similar. We have adopted the approach of treating the animals for both infection and rejection when we believe the

pigs are manifesting lethargy, anorexia, fever or coughing. Housing of the animals can also present a problem. Swine, particularly the domestic swine, require a great deal of space to grow adequately. Care of the animals is also challenging in that the animals require weight dosed daily medications and close monitoring of their clinical status. Care provision is aided by assistance from well educated and informed animal care handlers. However, the clinical researcher must play a large role in the day to day assessment of the postoperative lung transplant animals.

Another pitfall of previous and current models of lung transplantation is the issue of whether we are adequately investigating appropriate parameters of function and development of the transplanted lungs. Major influences on transplanted lungs include denervation, long-term immunosuppression and chronic rejection. Functional changes that occur as a result of these influences have recently been reported.[28–32] Functional and morphologic changes measured in animal models of lung transplantation are possibly a reflection of underlying physiologic changes at the subcellular level which have not yet been fully explored. To date, our relatively gross functional and developmental evaluations of transplanted lungs and lobes may not be getting to the basis of these changes. In future studies, we must examine functional activity at the cellular and subcellular level to help us better understand the overall functional and developmental changes that are occurring in experimental transplanted lungs.

REFERENCES

1. Metras H. Note preliminaire sur la greffe totale du poumon chez le chein. C R Acad Sci (Paris) 1950; 231:1176-8.
2. Hardy JD, Alican F. Lung transplantation. Adv Surg 1966; 2:235-64.
3. Neptune WB. Experimental lung transplantation. J Thorac Surg 1953; 26:275-89.
4. Byers JM, Sabanayagam P, Baker RR, Hutchins GM. Pathologic changes in baboon lung allografts. Ann Surg 1973; 178:754-60.

5. Haglin JJ, Arner O. Physiologic studies of the baboon living on only the reimplanted lung. Surg Forum 1964; 15:175-6.

6. Nakae S, Wells WR, Theodorides T, Sugg WL. Respiratory function following cardiopulmonary denervation in dog, cat and monkey. Surg Gynecol Obstet 1967; 125:1285-92.

7. Prop J, Wagenaar-Hilbers JPA, Peterson AH, Wildevuur CRH. Diagnosis of rejection in rat lung allografts by bronchoalveolar lavage. Transplant Proc 1987; 19:3779-80.

8. Prop J. Characteristics of cells lavaged from rejecting lung allografts in rats. Transplant Proc 1988; 20:217-8.

9. Hislop AA, Odom NJ, McGregor GA, Haworth SG. Growth potential of the immature transplanted lung. J Thorac Cardiovasc Surg 1990; 100:360-70.

10. Rendas A, Branthwaite M, Reid L. Growth of pulmonary circulation in normal pigs—structural analysis and cardiopulmonary function. J Appl Physio 1978; 45(5):806-17.

11. Crombleholme TM, Adzick NS, Hardy K et al. Pulmonary lobar transplantation in neonatal swine: a model for treatment of congenital diaphragmatic hernia. J Pediatr Surg 1990; 25(1):11-8.

12. Crombleholme TM, Adzick NS, Longaker MT et al. Reduced-size lung transplantation in neonatal swine: technique and short term physiologic response. Ann Thorac Surg 1990; 49:55-60.

13. Jennings RW, Lorenz HP, Duncan BW et al. Adult-to-neonate lung transplantation: anatomic considerations. J Pediatr Surg 1992; 10:1285-90.

14. Backer CL, Ohtake S, Zales VR et al. Living related lobar lung transplantation in beagle puppies. J Pediatr Surg 1991; 26:429-33.

15. Wain JC, Suen HC, Donahue DM, Ryan DP. Lobar lung allografts: acute studies with an elevated native pulmonary vascular resistance. Surg Forum 1991; XLII:415-7.

16. Ryan DP, Suen HC, Doody DP, Donahue DM, Wain JC. Neonatal heterotopic reduced-volume lung transplantation for congenital diaphragmatic hernia. Surg Forum 1992; XLIII:621-3.

17. Lillehei CW, Everts E, Shamberger RC. Reduced-size lung transplantation from adult to neonatal sheep. J Pediatr Surg 1992; 27:1153-6.

18. Furchgott RF, Zawadzki JV. The obligatory role of endothelial cells in the relaxation of arterial smooth muscle by acetylcholine. Nature 1980; 288:373-6.

19. Johns RA, Peach MJ, Flanagan TL, Kron IL. Probing of the canine internal mammary artery damages endothelium and impairs vasodilation due to prostacyclin and endothelium-derived relaxing factor. J Thorac Cardiovasc Surg 1989; 97(2):252-8.

20. Schele W. A simple method for volumetry of organs in quantitative stereology. Mikroskopie 1970; 26:57.

21. J. Gil. Models of Lung Disease. New York: Marcel Dekker, Inc., 1990.

22. Dunnill MS. Quantitative methods in the study of pulmonary pathology. Thorax 1962; 17:320-8.

23. Weibel ER, Gomez DM. A principle for counting tissue structures on random sections. J Appl Physiol 1962; 17:343-8.

24. Thomas DD, Standaert TA, Anton WF, Jones DR, Godwin JD, Hodson WA, Allen MD. Growth potential of the transplanted lung in the infant primate. Abstract. 29th Meeting, Society of Thoracic Surgeons. January 25-27, 1993.

25. Cowan CSM, Staub NC, Edmunds LH. Changes in the fluid compartments and dry weights of reimplanted dog lungs. J Appl Physiol 1976; 40:962-70.

26. Pearce ML, Yamashita J, Beazell J. Measurement of pulmonary edema. Circ Res 1965; 16:482-9.

27. Gomez RA, Sturgill BC, Chevalier RL, Boyd DG, Lessard JL, Owens GK, Peach MJ. Fetal expression of muscle-specific isoactins in multiple organs of the Wistar-Kyoto rat. Cell Tissue Res 1987; 250:7-12.

28. Johnson AM, Teague WG, Barone GW et al. Decreased vascular compliance after reimplantation of the left lower lobe in young pigs. Surg Forum 1988; XXXIX:288-9.

29. McGahren ED, Teague WG, Flanagan TL et al. Airway obstruction following autologous

reimplantation of the porcine lobe. J Thorac Cardiovasc Surg 1989; 97(4):587-91.

30. Hobson C, Teague WG, Tribble CG et al. Denervation of transplanted porcine lung causes airway obstruction. Ann Thorac Surg 1991; 52:1295-9.

31. Kern JA, Chan BK, Flanagan TL, Tribble CG, Kron IL. Long-term function of reduced-size porcine lobar pulmonary transplants: studies of vascular compliance. Ann Thorac Surg, 1992; 53(4):583-9.

32. Chan BK, Kern JA, Flanagan TL, Tribble CG, Kron IL: Effects of in vivo cyclosporine administration on responses of isolated vascular segments. Circ Suppl 1992; 86(5):II-295-II-299.

FUNCTION AND GROWTH POTENTIAL OF EXPERIMENTAL REDUCED-SIZE LUNG TRANSPLANTS

John A. Kern

INTRODUCTION

Successful reduced-size lung transplantation is predicated on the ability to dissect, preserve and reimplant an isolated pulmonary lobe or segment as a single whole lung. Reduced-size lung transplantation implies that the donor, whether cadaveric or living related, is larger than the recipient with the recipient most likely a child or young adult with a small thoracic cage. As for most organ and tissue transplantation the foundation for clinical reduced-size lung transplantation was built in the research laboratory and began as early as the 1940s.

Demikhov, a Russian physiologist, was able to successfully autotransplant individual pulmonary lobes in dogs as early as 1947. C. E. Huggins in 1959 reported the experimental reimplantation of isolated left lower lobes in dogs by successfully suturing the divided vessels and bronchus.[1] Previous experiments usually focused on whole lung reimplantation and rarely did such studies document long-term survival.[2-5] In 1966 Yeh and his colleagues reported successful experimental lobar reimplantation in dogs and were the first to suggest, based on functional results, that "from the standpoint of procurement and surgical mortality,

Reduced-size Lung Transplantation, edited by John A. Kern, M.D. and Irving L. Kron, M.D.; © 1993 R.G. Landes Company.

the use of single lobes may be preferable to whole lungs when clinical transplantation becomes a reality."[6]

While improved transplant techniques and enhanced immunosuppression have clearly enabled successful whole lung transplantation to become a reality, isolated lobar transplants have recently been viewed as a potential treatment modality for some children with otherwise incurable end-stage lung disease. The clinical experience with reduced-size lung transplantation is limited and most data which have appeared describing function of reduced-size lung transplants have been gathered from experimental models.[7-13] Until long-term survivors of clinical reduced-size lung transplantation can be studied, we need to critically review the experimental literature to help guide our clinical practices.

While most early studies of experimental lung transplantation were survival studies, many of today's experiments utilize meticulous invasive monitoring techniques which thoroughly evaluate all aspects of the transplanted lung's physiology. Some of these techniques were reviewed in Chapter 4. While most reports of reduced-size lung transplantation have been studies of early graft function, a few chronic studies have been done. This chapter will review studies of pulmonary vascular physiology, airway mechanics, gas exchange and growth potential of experimental reduced-size lung transplants. Study methods will be described, data will be interpreted and clinical significance and limitations will be discussed.

PULMONARY VASCULAR RESISTANCE

BACKGROUND

Childhood lung diseases which are potentially treatable through reduced-size lung transplantation include primary pulmonary hypertension, pulmonary atresia and congenital heart disease with resulting Eisenmenger-type physiology. In each of these conditions, native pulmonary vascular resistance is very high. One goal of transplantation is to provide a graft with a compliant pulmonary vascular bed capable of accepting the majority of the cardiac output.

Increases in blood flow through a healthy adult pulmonary vascular bed are accompanied by capillary recruitment and vasodilation which result in a fall in pulmonary vascular resistance and maintenance of the pulmonary artery pressure.[7,14,15] This response is known to occur in man and in commonly studied animals such as adult dogs and pigs.[7] In *neonatal* swine, however, increases in flow through an otherwise normal pulmonary vascular bed result in a significant *rise* in pulmonary vascular resistance and pulmonary artery pressure, with a resultant fall in cardiac output.[15] It is believed that the *immature* pulmonary vascular bed of the young pig, and possibly of the human, is already fully recruited and maximally dilated with no further ability to accommodate increases in flow.[7]

These functional findings are further appreciated by reviewing morphologic studies done by Reid and colleagues who studied growth of the pulmonary circulation in the normal pig and correlated it with human lung growth.[16] They found that intra-acinar arterial extension and structural remodeling is not complete in the pig until approximately 12 weeks of age and in man not until 11 years. In addition, functional studies in human infants with normal lungs and no pre-existing heart disease indicate a limited ability of the immature lung to modulate pulmonary vascular resistance in response to acute hypoxia. This limitation is not seen in adults.[17] It is likely that structural remodeling and maturation occurring in the immature lung have few functional effects during the basal resting state and are only apparent when determining the reserve capacity of the lung under certain stress conditions such as increases in pulmonary blood flow. Such conditions would likely be encountered by a lung allograft placed into a neonate with congenital diaphragmatic hernia and severe pulmonary hypoplasia. These background data concerning lung development would suggest that mature lung tissue might be superior to immature lung tissue when the need for neonatal or pediatric lung transplantation arises. A considerable amount of experimental research has been done examining this issue.

ACUTE STUDIES OF PULMONARY VASCULAR RESISTANCE

The first studies to appear which reported on the acute changes in pulmonary vascular resistance following experimental reduced-size lobar transplantation were from the University of California San Francisco's Fetal Treatment Program.[7,18] In 1990 Crombleholme and his associates reported the results of studies in which they transplanted the left lower lobe of 20 kg pigs into the left chest cavity of 6–8 kg piglets. In these acute hemodynamic studies, electromagnetic flow transducers were positioned around the main pulmonary artery and left pulmonary artery of the recipients for continuous measurements of cardiac output and flow distribution to the right and left

(reduced-size transplant) lungs prior to and after transplantation. Left atrial and pulmonary artery pressures were monitored continuously with indwelling catheters and a constricting tourniquet was placed around the right pulmonary artery in order to simulate clinical conditions of high native pulmonary vascular resistance and preferentially shunt blood through the transplanted lobe (Fig. 1). Pulmonary vascular resistance (PVR) was calculated using the formula:

$$\text{PVR (dynes} \times s \times cm^{-5}) = \text{pulmonary artery pressure (mm Hg)} - \text{left atrial pressure (mm Hg)/cardiac output (mL/s)} \times 1332.^{7}$$

Hemodynamic measurements were recorded before and after transplantation of

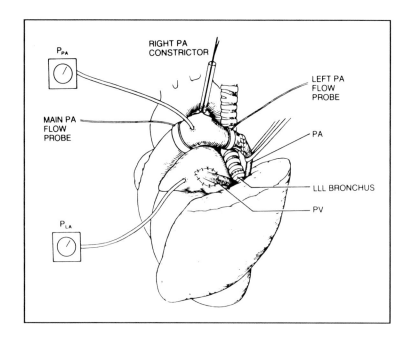

Fig. 1. Experimental design demonstrating evaluation of pulmonary hemodynamics of a porcine reduced-size lung transplant. Flow probes are placed around the pulmonary arteries and indwelling catheters are used to measure pressure. A tourniquet is placed around the right pulmonary artery to divert the entire cardiac output to the reduced-size transplant. (Reproduced with permission from W.B. Saunders and the Journal of Pediatric Surgery.)

the reduced-size left lower lobe, first with the right pulmonary artery open and then with the right pulmonary artery occluded to preferentially shunt blood to the transplanted reduced-size lobe.

These investigators were the first to report that a lobar graft from a more mature donor transplanted into a younger recipient as a single lung was technically feasible and hemodynamically well tolerated.[7] Acutely, the reduced-size lobar transplant functioned well and displayed acceptable hemodynamics over the short term of the study period, which lasted up to four hours. Left atrial and pulmonary artery pressures were not altered after the reduced-size transplant procedure and relative flow to the right and left sides was similar pre- and posttransplant. These results indicated adequate vascular capacity of the more mature lobe to accommodate the basal resting cardiac output of the neonatal recipient.[7] An unusual finding was the dramatic rise in pulmonary vascular resistance in the transplanted reduced-size lobe following occlusion of the contralateral pulmonary artery. Pulmonary vascular resistance rose from 864 (dyne x s x cm^{-5}) to 2,934 upon shunting the entire cardiac output through the lobar graft.[7] While this acute rise in pulmonary vascular resistance in the reduced-size transplant was no worse than that seen in the normally innervated native immature whole left lung, such significant rises in PVR may not be well tolerated in clinical reduced-size transplants.

It is possible that the vascular response in this model was due to a limited ability of the acutely denervated reduced-size lobe to modulate pulmonary vascular resistance acutely and that this response to denervation would resolve over time.[7] However, the donor animals in this study were only 20 kg pigs and although they were more mature than the recipients, they were far from adult and lung maturation would not have been complete. An alternative explanation, which was discounted by the investigators, is that the rise in PVR in the reduced-size transplants after occluding the contralateral pulmonary artery was due to immaturity of the pulmonary vascular bed of the *not fully mature* lobar transplants. In addition, this abnormal vascular reactivity or "acute denervation response" of transplanted immature porcine lobes does *not* resolve over time as was demonstrated in an earlier study in a similar model.[14]

Johnson et al[14] reimplanted the isolated left lower lobes in 20 kg piglets (the same size as the donors in Crombleholme's study) and after 10 weeks of additional recipient somatic growth (final body weight approximately 80 kg) occluded the contralateral pulmonary artery. Pulmonary artery pressure and pulmonary vascular resistance still rose abnormally in the reimplanted lobes, even after the additional posttransplant somatic growth and maturation. This abnormal rise in resistance and pressure was not seen in normally innervated nonreimplanted lobes.[14] Pulmonary vascular resistance (with the contralateral pulmonary artery occluded) was 12.7 ± 3.9 (mmHg/L/min) in the transplanted immature lobes and only 4.4 ± 0.5 in the control lobes ($p < 0.05$). Therefore, while the initial report by Crombleholme demonstrated that reduced-size lung transplantation is technically feasible, it also revealed a potential limitation if fully mature lobes are not used for the reduced-size transplant.

Acute studies of pulmonary vascular function of experimental living related reduced-size lung transplants have also been reported by Wain and his colleagues from Boston.[12] These investigators have been using the lamb model and in 1991 reported the acute function of heterotopically transplanted reduced-size lung transplants with an elevated native pulmonary vascular resistance.[12] Pulmonary vascular resistance and pulmonary artery pressure were measured in fully mature right upper lobes which had been transplanted heterotopically from adult ewes into the left chest of young lambs. Ultrasonic flow probes were used to measure total cardiac output and differential blood flow to the right (native) and left (transplanted) lungs. Pulmonary artery, graft pulmonary vein and left atrial pressures were measured with indwelling catheters. After reventilation of the reduced-size graft, the recipient's right pulmonary artery was ligated *distal to the native right upper lobe branches* and the bronchus intermedius was clamped. This is an important technical maneuver because it resulted in a preparation which preferentially increased flow not only through the reduced-size mature lobar transplant on the left, but also through the native immature right upper lobe. The results of this elegant study are very important. While pulmonary vascular resistance (measured in Wood units) was similar in the native immature right lung and the reduced-size transplant prior to clamping the right pulmonary artery (13 ± 4 vs. 23 ± 6 respectively), PVR rose significantly in the native right upper lobe after clamping but remained *normal in the reduced-size transplant* (71 ± 56 vs. 24 ± 9 respectively). Over the course of the four-hour study period, PVR remained elevated in the native right upper lobe but stayed normal in the reduced-size mature lobar graft (60 ± 38 vs. 33 ± 15 respectively).[12]

The key feature in this study is that the transplanted reduced-size lobes were harvested from adult animals and therefore had fully developed vascular beds which allowed for adequate capillary recruitment in response to increased flow. This is in contrast to Crombleholme's study in which more mature, but not completely mature lobes were used for transplantation into neonatal piglets; although the pig lobes functioned well, they were unable to fully accommodate an increased blood flow without exhibiting a rise in pulmonary vascular resistance. The difference in these two acute studies is likely a result of the degree of lung maturity of the lobar transplant. From these data, it might be recommended that reduced-size lung transplants in humans utilize *fully mature lobes.*

CHRONIC STUDIES OF PULMONARY VASCULAR RESISTANCE

Backer and his colleagues reported in 1991 a series of living related reduced-size lung transplants in beagle puppies.[9] These investigators harvested the left lower lobes from fully mature beagles and transplanted them into beagle puppies. Although this chronic study demonstrated that long-term survival following experimental reduced-size lung transplantation is possible, no objective data were quantified. These investigators did, however, perform pulmonary angiograms on the long-term survivors. Ten of the 20 recipient animals died within 50 days of transplant and prior to angiographic analysis. The causes of death in these animals were rejection in four animals, infection in three animals and bronchial dehiscence in three animals. Of the 10 surviving puppies that were studied angiographically, 2 were found to have normal angiograms, 5 had diminished blood flow to the left lower lobe transplant and 3 had complete left pulmonary artery occlusion.[9] While no objective data concerning long-term pulmonary vascular reactivity of the reduced-size lobar transplants were reported, one animal with angiographically normal graft blood flow underwent balloon occlusion of the contralateral right pulmonary artery and survived for two days.[9] The cause of death in this animal was not made clear. This study was the first to indicate the ability of a reduced-size lung transplant to solely support life.

In another study out of the University of California San Francisco's Fetal Treatment Laboratory, reduced-size lung transplantation was again performed in neonatal piglets.[8] In these experiments the donor lung tissue was the left upper lobe apical segment and the donors were adult pigs of up to 60 kg. The recipient neonatal piglets weighed 5–8 kg. The recipient piglets were allowed to recover and 5 of 10 animals survived for more than one week.[8] During the second postoperative week pulmonary blood flow was analyzed by placing ultrasonic flow probes around the aorta and the left (reduced-size graft) pulmonary artery. In two animals that survived to final analysis the ratio of right to left pulmonary artery blood flow was reported as 1:1.3, with the higher ratio of blood flow going to the reduced-size transplant.[8] The reduced-size transplant presumably had a more compliant pulmonary vascular bed than the native immature contralateral lung.

A report in 1992 by Lillehei documented long-term survival of neonatal lambs after receiving reduced-size lobar transplants from nonrelated adult sheep.[13] This study included evidence of *normal* perfusion of the allograft lobe at 10 days to two weeks posttransplant but no other hemodynamic parameters were reported.[13]

Recent studies from the University of Virginia have focused particularly on long-term function of reduced-size lung transplants and have also utilized a porcine model.[10] Studies of pulmonary vascular resistance have been performed approximately three months following transplantation of mature left lower lobes from adult pigs with a mean weight of 109 kg (n = 10) into nine week old piglets with a mean weight of 20 kg. The donor animals in these studies were sexually mature six to seven month old animals with functionally mature lungs.

Following the transplant procedure the recipients were allowed to recover for at least 12 weeks and increased their body weight approximately four-fold to 83 kg. Of 10 piglets undergoing transplant, five ultimately survived for complete analysis of pulmonary vascular resistance. With the animals intubated and the sternum opened, pulmonary hemodynamics of the reduced-size transplants were measured with indwelling pulmonary artery catheters.[10] Cardiac output and pulmonary blood flow measurements were made with a thermistor-tipped Swan-Ganz catheter using the thermodilution technique. Measurements were taken in the resting state and then with the right pulmonary artery totally occluded with atraumatic vascular clamps in order to increase flow through the graft. Results from these experiments are shown in Table 1. As controls, age and size matched adult animals underwent evaluation of the native innervated left lower lobes acutely following left upper lobectomy. Results were also compared to transplanted immature left lower lobes in animals which

Table 1. Long-term Hemodynamics of Porcine Reduced-size Mature Lobar Lung Transplants

	Pulmonary Artery Pressure (mmHg)		Pulmonary Vascular Resistance (mmHg/L/Min)	
	Pre	Post	Pre	Post
Reduced-size (mature) Transplants	31 ± 2	49 ± 2	2.1 ± 0.4	5.4 ± 0.9
Immature Lobar Transplants	25 ± 3	60 ± 13	2.6 ± 0.3[a]	12.9 ± 3.9[a,b]
Control Adult Lobes	27 ± 2	46 ± 3	1.6 ± 0.2	4.0 ± 0.6

[a]p<0.05 versus control adult lobes
[b]p<0.05 versus reduced-size transplants
Pre=before clamping the contralateral pulmonary artery; Post=after clamping the contralateral pulmonary artery.

were also allowed to recover for 12 weeks. Pulmonary artery pressure and pulmonary vascular resistance were similar in all three groups prior to clamping the right pulmonary artery. Upon shunting the entire cardiac output through the isolated left lower lobe, the reduced-size mature lobar transplants responded in a fashion similar to the normally innervated mature control left lower lobes (PVR postclamp = 5.4 ± 0.9 mmHg/L/ min in the reduced-size grafts vs. 4.0 ± 0.6 mmHg/L/min in the control adult lobes and 12.9 ± 3.9 in the transplanted immature lobes.) The reduced-size transplants were able to accommodate the increased blood flow without an abnormal rise in pulmonary vascular resistance or pulmonary artery pressure.[10] Under the controlled experimental conditions of the study the mature lobar transplants appeared capable of supporting the animal.[10]

A limitation of this study, as with most chronic studies of experimental lung transplantation, is that the animals were allowed to recover, survive and grow with a normal contralateral lung. In addition, at the time of final lung analysis during the period of contralateral lung exclusion, all of the animals were mechanically ventilated and breathing 100% oxygen. The ability of a reduced-size lung transplant to support life and sustain growth of a recipient with a nonfunctioning contralateral lung is unknown at the present time.

AIRWAY FUNCTION AND PULMONARY MECHANICS

In addition to adequate reactivity of the pulmonary vascular bed, the transplanted reduced-size lung must also provide adequate airway function. In cases of unilateral reduced-size lung transplantation for congenital diaphragmatic hernia with severe pulmonary hypoplasia, for example, the native underdeveloped lung would have poor ventilatory compliance and ventilation would be preferentially directed toward the reduced-size graft. The graft needs to be compliant

enough with adequate airway resistance to allow preferential ventilation to occur. Although not extensively studied, a few reports have appeared which have examined static and dynamic compliance and resistance of experimental reduced-size lung transplants both acutely and chronically.

A study by Crombleholme measured the static and dynamic compliance and resistance of reduced-size left lower lobe transplants for a period of up to two hours posttransplant.[7] A porcine model was used and donor left lower lobes were harvested from 20 kg animals and transplanted into 6–8 kg piglets. Compliance and resistance of the isolated reduced-size transplants and of the normal contralateral right lungs were measured by preferentially intubating the bronchus of the lung to be studied and connecting the endobronchial tube to a Puritan-Bennett (Los Angeles, CA) model 7200 ventilator.[7] Tidal volumes were 10 to 15 ml/kg and the respiratory rate was adjusted to maintain normal arterial blood gas values as determined on a commercial blood gas analyzer. During the measurements the lungs were ventilated with 100% oxygen. The results of this acute study indicated that the reduced-size left lower lobe grafts were preferentially ventilated when compared to the native right lungs of the young recipient animals.[7] Static compliance of the reduced-size transplants was significantly higher than in the native immature right lung. Static compliance was 5.5 ± 0.2 ml/ cm in the native right lungs and 8.2 ± 0.3 ml/ cm in the reduced-size transplants (p < 0.001). Dynamic compliance was 5.6 ± 0.2 ml/cm in the native right lungs and 6.2 ± 0.3 ml/cm in the reduced-size grafts.[7] The superior compliance of the transplanted reduced-size lobes was presumably due to "continued alveolarization during the pulmonary growth and development of the more mature lobar donor."[7] The more mature lobar graft likely had a higher number of respiratory alveoli per unit lung volume, which resulted in compliance superior to that of the immature native right lung.[7–19]

Airway resistance was not significantly different between the reduced-size transplants and the native immature right lungs. Resistance was 22.3 ± 2.5 cm H_2O/L/s in the native right lungs and 21.8 ± 1.3 cm H_2O/L/s in the reduced-size grafts.[7] These findings are perhaps a bit unusual because we would expect the airways to be larger in the more mature lobar transplants, which should provide lower resistance to airflow. Perhaps the acute response to denervation or the trauma of cold immersion resulted in bronchoconstriction which was slow to resolve in the reduced-size transplant.

A recent report from our laboratory at the University of Virginia described chronic studies of dynamic resistance and compliance of reduced-size mature lobar transplants.[20] Mature left lower lobes from adult pigs were transplanted into 18 to 20 kg piglets at nine weeks of age. The recipients were allowed to recover for 12 weeks during which time their body weight increased four-fold. To serve as a control, a second group of nine week old piglets underwent left thoracotomy and left upper lobectomy. The left lower lobes in these animals were not manipulated and were subject to compensatory growth over the course of the 12 week growth period. At the time of final study the pigs were anesthetized, intubated and mechanically ventilated. Isolated measurements of the right or left lung were made after occluding the contralateral airways with intrabronchial balloon catheters positioned bronchoscopically.[20] Airflow and transrespiratory pressure were measured at the airway opening using a pneumotachometer and two differential pressure transducers as described in Chapter 4. Signals were digitized at a rate of 15 ms with a data acquisition system and stored on diskettes. Gas flow and transrespiratory pressure were recorded over 10 ventilated breaths. Pressure-volume loops were constructed for each breath by hand editing the three points of zero flow with a manual cursor and text editor. Dynamic pulmonary compliance was calculated as the slope of the line of best fit through the origin and apex of the pressure-volume relationship. Dynamic airway resistance was calculated from measurements of

the total pressure change at 50% tidal volume divided by the absolute value of flow at that volume.[20]

In this chronic study, dynamic compliance of the reduced-size transplants was lower than in the native right lungs and was also lower than the compliance of normally innervated left lower lobes of the control animals.[20] Compliance in the native right lungs of animals receiving a reduced-size allograft was 27.6 ± 2.5 ml/cm. Compliance of the reduced-size grafts was 18.4 ± 1.7 ml/cm versus 24.9 ± 1.6 ml/cm in the normal left lower lobes of nontransplanted animals after compensatory growth ($p < 0.05$).[20] Dynamic airway resistance, however, was normal in the reduced-size transplants (5.3 ± 1.4 cm/L/s in the reduced-size grafts vs. 5.4 ± 0.7 cm/L/s in the contralateral right lungs). Normal airway resistance of the reduced-size transplants, we believe, was due to the fact that the lobes were fully mature with completely developed distal airways at the time of transplantation. Histologic evaluation of the reduced-size grafts revealed normal appearing architecture and normal size distal airways (Fig. 2).

Compliance, however, was abnormal in the transplanted mature lobes and this could not be explained by the effects of thoracotomy, pleural adhesions or immunosuppressive therapy as the control animals also underwent thoracotomy, had similar degrees of adhesions and received similar drug therapy yet had normal compliance. It is likely that the abnormal compliance was a result of progressive loss of elastic recoil of the pulmonary parenchyma perhaps due to fibrosis resulting from chronic low grade rejection. This has not been proven, however, and clearly would not be apparent in acute studies which demonstrate normal pulmonary compliance of reduced-size lung transplants.

GAS EXCHANGE

Most studies of reduced-size lung transplants, whether acute or chronic, have included data on gas exchange provided by the graft.[7,10,21] Indeed, such data are important as

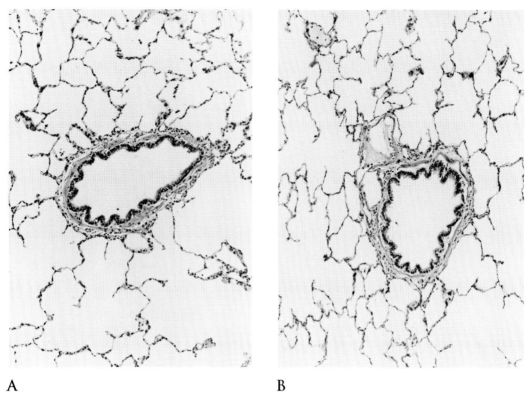

A   B

Fig. 2. Histologic sections of: (A) reduced-size porcine lung transplant three months after transplant and (B) normal porcine lung. Normal airway size and pulmonary architecture of the reduced-size transplant is evident. (H and E stain; 125 x magnification prior to reproduction.)

all other functions of the lung are secondary to its ability to oxygenate and ventilate. Rather than review this extensive subset of data, it will suffice to say that most studies reporting these parameters of lung function have demonstrated adequate oxygenation and ventilation through the reduced-size transplant. In fact, in some acute studies such as those from the University of California San Francisco, the superior compliance of the reduced-size graft as compared to the native right lung resulted in preferential ventilation of the graft and a profound respiratory alkalosis of blood coming from the graft.[7] Chronic studies from our own laboratory have not demonstrated this phenomenon, but ventilation has been uniformly adequate when assessed by way of selective pulmonary vein blood sampling and by systemic arterial blood gas analysis with the

contralateral lung excluded.[10] Oxygenation acutely has been documented by several investigators as being excellent. Chronically, while still adequate, oxygenation is somewhat diminished. Studies from our laboratory have documented adequate oxygenation through the reduced-size transplant with the animal breathing supplemental oxygen as well as room air.[10]

GROWTH POTENTIAL OF REDUCED-SIZE TRANSPLANTS

To date only one experimental study has been reported which examined the growth potential of reduced-size lung transplants.[11] This is a very critical issue. To provide adequate long-term function after transplantation into a child, reduced-size lung transplants, it would seem, need to undergo compensatory growth in proportion with the recipient's somatic growth. Without some degree of compensatory growth the transplanted reduced-size lobe could only be used as a temporary measure, providing pulmonary support until the recipient either matures a contralateral hypoplastic lung (in which case the graft could be removed) or outgrows the reduced-size transplant and is of large enough size to receive a second allograft, either a whole lung or another lobe. Clinical evidence suggests that young children are capable of compensatory lung growth up to the age of five years.[22] This compensatory growth is of normally innervated developing pulmonary tissue not exposed to the effects of immunosuppression and chronic rejection. Individuals between the ages of 6 and 20 years have some ability to increase lung volumes after partial lung resections, however, it is unclear as to whether this results from true hyperplasia and compensatory growth or from simple hypertrophy.[22] In adults this ability is limited. It appears, based on clinical data, that the ability for compensatory lung growth gradually disappears with age.[22] Because it is not known what factors are responsible for compensatory lung growth in children, it is not known whether already mature reduced-size lung transplants, when grafted into a young child, will display any increase in functional capacity as the host grows.

The one experimental attempt to address the issue of growth of reduced-size lung transplants was performed in our laboratory.[11] Mature left lower lobes were harvested from adult pigs weighing 105 kg and were transplanted into nine week old piglets (n=6) with a mean weight of 22 kg. The piglets were allowed to grow for three months at the end of which time they weighed 85 kg. *As controls, left lower lobes from pigs of similar age and size as the donors* were evaluated in a similar fashion.[11] Parameters assayed were lung weight and water content, fixed volume, functional residual capacity, alveolar size and number, and alveolar airspace volume percent.[11] In this study, gross parameters of lobar growth were not terribly revealing. However, fixed volume and lobar weight *were* increased in the transplanted mature lobes compared to the control lobes. More importantly, however, functional and morphologic assessment of lobar growth revealed *no* increase in functional residual capacity of the reduced-size transplants (as determined by helium dilution) and *no* increase in total number of alveoli. Functional residual capacity of the transplanted mature lobes was 600 ± 40 ml after three additional months of growth whereas FRC was 606 ± 100 ml in the control lobes.[11] Total alveolar number was $107.4 \times 10^6 \pm 16$ in the reduced-size transplants and $95.1 \times 10^6 \pm 10.7$ in the control lobes.[11] Alveolar size was similar between the two groups and alveolar air space volume percent was *decreased* in the transplanted lobes. These findings indicate that, at least in the pig, any growth (as reflected in increased weight and fixed volume) of the reduced-size transplant was likely a result of an increase in connective tissue and cellular components of the lung and not a result of an increase in alveolar number or size.[11] Obviously, this type of nonfunctional compensatory growth is less than ideal for the pediatric patient receiving a reduced-size mature lobar transplant. We do not know how this lack of functional growth will impact on the host and whether the same will hold true in human reduced-size lung transplants.

SUMMARY

Experimental studies of reduced-size lung transplants have been ongoing for several years. Because clinical experience is so severely limited we need to be guided in our clinical practice by what we are learning in the research laboratory and use experimental data to help guide the future of reduced-size lung transplantation. Nevertheless, we need to be aware of the limitations of these experimental models. Most studies have been acute in nature and although they establish the feasibility and adequate early function of such transplants they do not provide long-term data. On the other hand, the few long-term studies which have been done are limited by the fact that all animals survived over the long-term with normal contralateral lungs. This would not be the case in clinical reduced-size lung transplantation. Unfortunately, long-term models of reduced-size lung transplants are difficult to establish and are costly. Attempts are ongoing to establish a model of reduced-size lung transplantation in which the recipient either undergoes a staged contralateral pneumonectomy or gradual ablation of the contralateral lung through occlusion of the hilar structures. Mortality in these studies is likely to be high and data have yet to appear. In general, experimental reduced-size lung transplants are feasible and appear sound from a physiologic standpoint. Pulmonary vascular function and responsiveness of these transplants are adequate for the young recipients *when fully mature lobes are used.* Airway function and pulmonary mechanics are also acceptable both acutely and long-term. Oxygenation and ventilation through the reduced-size grafts do not seem to be a problem. Growth potential, however, may be an issue. More research is needed to help resolve these issues and allow reliable and predictable reduced-size lung transplantation become more of a clinical reality.

REFERENCES

1. Huggins CE. Reimplantation of lobes of the lung, an experimental technique. The Lancet 1959; 2:1059-62.

2. Juvenelle AA, Citret C, Wiles CE et al. Pneumonectomy with replantation of the lung in the dog for physiologic study. J Thorac Surg 1951; 21:111-13.

3. Davis, HA, O'Connor JP, Coloviras GJ, Strawn DL. Homologous transplantation of the lung. Arch Surg 1952; 64:745-51.

4. Neptune WB, Redondo HB, Bailey CP. Surg Forum 1953; 379-81.

5. Borrie J, Montgomerie. Proc Univ Otago Med Sch. 1958; 36:9-10

6. Yeh JTT, Manning H, Ellison LT, Ellison RG. Anatomic and physiologic consideration in pulmonary lobar reimplantation. Surg Forum 1966; 17:211-13.

7. Crombleholme TM, Adzick NS, Hardy K et al. Pulmonary lobar transplantation in neonatal swine: a model for treatment of congenital diaphragmatic hernia. J Pediatr Surg 1990; 25(1):11-18.

8. Jennings RW, Lorenz HP, Duncan BW et al. Adult-to-neonate lung transplantation: anatomic considerations. J Pediatr Surg 1992; 10:1285-90.

9. Backer CL, Ohtake S, Zales VR, LoCicero III J, Michaelis LL, Idriss FS. Living related lobar lung transplantation in beagle puppies. J Pediatr Surg 1991; 26(4):429-33.

10. Kern JA, Tribble CG, Chan BBK, Flanagan TL, Kron IL. Reduced-size porcine lung transplantation: long-term studies of pulmonary vascular resistance. Ann Thorac Surg 1992; 53:583-9.

11. Kern JA, Tribble CG, Flanagan TL et al. Growth potential of porcine reduced-size mature pulmonary lobar transplants. J Thorac Cardiovasc Surg 1992; 104:1329-32.

12. Wain JC, Suen HC, Donahue DM, Ryan DP. Lobar lung allografts: acute studies with an elevated native pulmonary vascular resistance. Surg Forum 1991; XLII:415-7.

13. Lillehei CW, Everts E, Shamberger RC. Reduced-size lung transplantation from adult to neonatal sheep. J Pediatr Surg 1992; 27(8):1153-6.

14. Johnson AM, Teague WG, Flanagan TL, McGahren ED, Kron IL. Decreased vascular compliance after reimplantation of the left lower lobe in young pigs. Ann Thorac Surg 1990; 50:277-80.

15. Crombleholme TM, Adzick NS, Longaker MT et al. Pulmonary vascular resistance in neonatal swine: response to right pulmonary artery occlusion, isoproterenol, and prostaglandin E1. J Pediatr Surg 1990; 25(8):861-6.

16. Rendas A, Branthwaite M, Reid L. Growth of pulmonary circulation in normal pig-structural and cardiopulmonary function. J Appl Physiol 1978; 45:806-17.

17. James LS, Rowe RD. The patten of response of pulmonary and systemic arterial

pressures in new born and older infants to short periods of hypoxia. J Pediat 1957; 51:5-11.

18. Crombleholme TM, Adzick NS, Longaker MT et al. Reduced-size lung transplantation in neonatal swine: technique and short term physiologic response. Ann Thorac Surg 1990; 49:55-60.

19. Hislop AA, Wigglesworth JS, Desai R: Alveolar development in the human fetus and infant. Early Human Development 1986; 13:1-11.

20. Kern JA, Tribble CG, Zografakis JG et al. Analysis of airway function of immature whole lung transplants versus mature lobar transplants. Ann Thorac Surg 1993;In press.

21. Ryan DP, Suen HC, Doody DP, Donahue DM, Wain JC. Neonatal heterotopic reduced-volume lung transplantation for congenital diaphragmatic hernia. Surg Forum 1992; 43:621-3.

22. Laros CD, Westermann CJJ. Dilatation, compensatory growth, or both after pneumonectomy during childhood and adolescence. J Thorac Cardiovasc Surg 1987; 93:570-6.

CHAPTER 6

THE IDEAL PEDIATRIC LUNG ALLOGRAFT: MATURE LOBE VERSUS IMMATURE WHOLE LUNG

John A. Kern

INTRODUCTION

For the pediatric patient with end-stage lung disease in need of transplantation there are two transplant options available. The conventional form of transplant therapy has been the transplantation of size matched immature whole lungs. In neonates and children under the age of 10 to 12 years, this requires transplantation of a lung which is not yet fully mature with respect to lung volumes, airway size, vessel size, alveolar number, and airway and vessel morphology. The effects of transplantation on these developmental parameters are not fully known. The second option, which is the main focus of this monograph, is reduced-size lung transplantation. This technique has only recently been described and is obviously appealing for it would help alleviate the pediatric donor lung shortage and it would allow for living related lung transplantation with its potential immunologic advantages.[1] Whether one of these options is superior to the other with respect to long-term graft function and host survival is not known.

Clinically successful pediatric lung transplantation, whether using immature whole lungs or reduced-size mature lobes has not been studied long enough to allow determination of the fate of the graft and host over a prolonged time. This chapter will review the experimental data which exist concerning long-term function and growth of immature whole lung and

Reduced-size Lung Transplantation, edited by John A. Kern, M.D. and Irving L. Kron, M.D.; © 1993 R.G. Landes Company.

reduced-size lung transplants in order to make predictions as to which one of these two options might be optimal for the pediatric lung transplant recipient. While review of the data points out differences between the two options, this review is in no way meant to persuade the reader to use one form of therapy over the other. The fact remains that there are currently far too few pediatric donor lungs available to meet present demand. Any acceptable organ, whether it be an immature whole lung or a reduced-size adult lobe should potentially be used if it is safe for both the recipient and donor and the indications for transplantation are acceptable. Clinical reduced-size lung transplantation is too new and immature whole lung transplantation is becoming increasingly successful so that neither form of therapy should be discounted at the present time on the basis of experimental data.

BACKGROUND

It is difficult to compare two treatment options when: 1) little is known about the long-term results of both options and 2) only one experimental study has been done directly comparing the two options. Nevertheless, enough anecdotal and circumstantial data exist so that one can come to some relatively sound conclusions concerning this issue.

Most of the experimental data evaluating the function of immature lung transplants and of reduced-size mature lobar transplants have been generated in our own laboratory at the University of Virginia.[2-7] Recently, many other investigators have become interested in experimental pediatric lung transplantation and have developed models of *immature* whole lung transplantation in order to study growth potential of the transplanted immature lung.[8-11] This is a critical issue, as adequate function of immature whole lung transplants over time is clearly going to be related to proper growth and maturation of the graft. Unfortunately, little functional data have been generated from these studies. In addition, so little is known about what regulates normal postnatal lung development that trying to assess factors in-

fluencing the growth of a *transplanted* immature lung may be almost impossible.

At the University of Virginia we have used the porcine model of pediatric lung transplantation for several reasons. First, we are very familiar with the long-term care and handling of this animal. The pig is particularly tolerant of thoracotomy and recovers quickly. The anatomy is ideal for lung transplant procedures and the animals seem to tolerate transplantation quite well with acceptable operative mortality rates. In addition, we are fortunate in that functional and morphologic analyses of porcine lung development have been previously investigated by other researchers and correlations with human postnatal lung development have been clearly outlined.[12] While the exact time course for postnatal lung development may not be known for all mammals, previous investigators have noted that "the Laws of Human Lung Development may apply generally to (all) mammalian lung."[12] As a result, this chapter will review studies in species other than just pigs and correlations to human lung development and pediatric lung transplantation will be made based on this premise.

PULMONARY VASCULAR RESISTANCE

The hilar denervation associated with pulmonary transplantation has been shown to have specific vascular effects. Acutely, the effect of denervation on pulmonary vascular resistance is to cause it to increase when blood flow through that lung is increased.[13,14] This effect of denervation is generally thought to be only transient, however, and over time the pulmonary vascular resistance of the denervated transplanted lung will return to normal. Indeed, in many experimental models of adult lung transplantation pulmonary vascular resistance has been found to be normal.[14-17] An important concept, however, is that these have been models of adult lung transplantation and the transplanted lungs were from adult animals.

The previous review of pulmonary vascular resistance of experimental reduced-size lung transplants (Chapter 5) demonstrated that when completely mature lobes are used for transplantation into young animals, pulmonary vascular resistance is normal in the allograft acutely and chronically.[4,18] Not only is pulmonary vascular resistance of the reduced-size transplant normal, but it is superior to the vascular reactivity of the native immature lung as demonstrated by Wain in his studies in lambs.[18]

There are very few studies which have examined the pulmonary vascular bed and its response to increases in blood flow in transplanted *immature* lungs. A study by Johnson from the University of Virginia in 1990 reported on the "decreased vascular compliance after reimplantation of the left lower lobe in young pigs."[3] This study reported that abnormal pulmonary vascular responses persist well beyond the immediate posttransplant period, and that even as long as 10 weeks after reimplantation of the immature left lower lobe abnormally high pulmonary vascular resistance develops in response to increases in blood flow through the graft.[3]

A follow-up study from our laboratory compared pulmonary vascular resistance of reduced-size *mature* lobar transplants to reimplanted *immature* left lower lobes after similar degrees of postoperative somatic growth of the recipient animals.[4] In this study we found that pulmonary vascular compliance, as measured by changes in pulmonary artery pressure and pulmonary vascular resistance caused by increasing flow through the graft, was superior in the reduced-size mature lobar transplants compared to the reimplanted immature lobes.[4] We believe that either denervation or the mechanical insults of excising and preserving an immature lung during a critical stage of postnatal growth and development results in long-term functional abnormalities within the vascular bed. Differences in pulmonary vascular reactivity between immature and reduced-size mature lung transplants may be related to the degree of pulmonary vascular maturation at the time of transplantation.[4] Another theory which might explain the differences between the immature and mature transplanted lung is that of classic denervation induced receptor up-regulation of vascular smooth muscle which is seen in the

immature lung but not in the mature lobe. This receptor up-regulation results in vasoconstriction in response to stressful stimuli such as increases in flow.[3] In humans, the pulmonary vascular bed is not fully mature until at least 10 years of age, and based on these experimental data transplantation of lungs or reduced-size lobes from donors older than this would in theory be unlikely to show long-term pulmonary vascular abnormalities. These data of pulmonary vascular resistance, therefore, would dictate the use of a reduced-size mature lobe rather than an immature lung for pediatric and neonatal lung transplantation due to the more developed vascular bed of the mature lobe.

AIRWAY FUNCTION AND PULMONARY MECHANICS

Normal adult lungs are naturally more compliant than immature lungs.[19] As normal lungs develop, the terminal bronchioli become respiratory bronchioli and there is an increase in number and size of alveoli. In addition, the number of respiratory alveoli per unit lung volume increases and these factors together result in increased pulmonary compliance of the mature as compared to immature lung.[19] Pulmonary compliance is a measure of the elastic recoil of the lung and is also affected by the physical properties of the lung parenchyma, the surface tension of the alveoli and the mechanical properties of the chest wall. Airway resistance is a direct measure of obstruction to airflow and is affected most by the diameter of the lobar, segmental and subsegmental airways. Abnormally small or obstructed airways resulting from either arrested development in an immature lung or abnormal bronchoconstriction or bronchiolitis obliterans would result in abnormally high dynamic resistance.

The earliest lung transplant studies from our laboratory were experiments which examined the long-term effects of reimplantation of the *immature* porcine lung on dynamic compliance and resistance. These studies showed that autologous reimplantation of the immature left lower lobe leads to long-term adverse changes in flow-dependent measurements of airway patency.[2] These changes may be due to alterations in bronchomotor regulation imposed by denervation of the immature lung or to abnormal posttransplant development of the distal bronchial tree which (as we subsequently found), is most likely.[6] Hobson, also from the University of Virginia, looked at long-term pulmonary mechanics of reimplanted and transplanted immature left lower lobes in young piglets.[20] Again the findings were that abnormal dynamic resistance and compliance were present in both the autografted and allografted *immature* lobes. The added insults of chronic rejection and immunosuppression in the allograft group had no additional detrimental effects on airway mechanics. The authors concluded that *denervation of the immature porcine lung leads to long-term abnormalities of airflow.*[20] In addition, these abnormalities to airflow were correlated with abnormally small distal airways which, as will be shown later, were most likely a result of abnormal small airway development following transplantation of the immature lung.[20] These findings would have great significance for the pediatric lung transplant patient and are made even more relevant when we examine studies of reduced-size mature lobar transplants in the same species.

A study by Crombleholme examining reduced-size lung transplants in pigs revealed that immediate posttransplant dynamic *compliance was superior to compliance in the native immature contralateral lung* and that resistance was similar to the native lung.[1] This was an acute study, however, and the results differ a bit from the results of a subsequent chronic study of porcine reduced-size lung transplants performed in our own laboratory.

We performed a set of experiments which to date is the only report of a direct comparison of reduced-size mature lobar transplants and transplanted immature whole lungs as would be used for pediatric lung transplantation.[7] In this study three groups of nine week old piglets were utilized. The first group underwent left thoracotomy and left upper lobectomy with the normally innervated left lower lobe remaining undisturbed. (This group of animals would therefore undergo, if possible, some degree of compensatory growth of the normally innervated developing left lower lobe.) The second group of animals received an immature whole left lung transplant from age and size matched immature animals. The third group of animals received a reduced-size mature left lower lobe from adult sexually mature pigs. All animals were allowed to grow for three months at which time they underwent evaluation of dynamic airway resistance, pulmonary compliance and functional residual capacity of the isolated transplanted lobes or lungs and of the nonoperated right lungs. Results from this study are presented in Table 1. Dynamic compliance and resistance were similar in all three groups in the nonoperated right lung. On the left side, however, *dynamic resistance was significantly elevated only in the immature whole lung transplants.*[7] Resistance was normal in the reduced-size mature lobar transplants. Dynamic compliance was reduced in all groups, perhaps to some degree as a result of the thoracotomy. However, compliance was most significantly reduced in both of the allograft groups. The etiology of this abnormal compliance is unknown, but may be related to chronic low level rejection.

The etiology of abnormal dynamic airway resistance in the immature porcine whole lung transplants may be explained by reviewing another study from our laboratory in which we examined, morphologically, the terminal airways of normal mature porcine left lower lobes, mature left lower lobes which had undergone compensatory growth following left upper lobectomy during early life, reduced-size mature left lower lobe transplants, immature left lower lobe autografts and immature left lower lobe allografts.[6] All animals were studied after a similar degree of postoperative somatic growth. For final analysis, the lobes were fixed through the airways with formalin and cross-sectional areas of terminal, noncartilaginous airways from the lung periphery were traced on a video monitor. The results are displayed in Table 2. Unlike the immature porcine lobe, transplantation of the mature porcine lobe as a reduced-size transplant did not result in abnormally small airways (Fig. 1). These results indicate that the small

Table 1. Compliance and Resistance of Reduced-size Lobar and Immature Whole Lung Transplants in Pigs

	Compliance (ml/cm)		Resistance (cm/L/sec)	
	Right	Left	Right	Left
Control Lobes	32.5 ± 3.0	24.9 ± 1.6	4.0 ± 0.7	2.7 ± 0.4[a]
Immature Lung Transplants	35.3 ± 3.0	15.9 ± 1.8[ab]	3.7 ± 1.0	11.9 ± 2.6[ab]
Reduced-size Transplants	27.6 ± 2.5	18.4 ± 1.7[b]	5.4 ± 0.7	5.3 ± 1.4

[a]$p<0.05$ right versus left [b]$p<0.05$ versus ipsilateral control

airways and abnormal airway resistance seen in *immature* porcine lung transplants are likely due to *impaired small airway development following transplantation* and not to denervation induced bronchoconstriction.[6] Again, these results lead us to suggest that a mature reduced-size lobe may be superior to an immature whole lung for pediatric lung transplantation.

GROWTH POTENTIAL

We reviewed in the preceding chapter the data concerning growth potential of experimental reduced-size mature lobar transplants.[6] It appears that in the porcine model, although fixed volume and weight of the transplanted mature lobe increase over time, functional capacity as measured with the helium dilution technique and total alveolar number do not increase after transplantation into a growing animal.[6] Recently, several investigators have attempted to address the issue of growth potential of *immature* transplanted whole lungs.[8–11] Transplantation of an immature lung requires that, depending on the age of the transplant, many aspects

Table 2. Cross Sectional Airway Area

Group	n	Airway Area (μm^2 x 10^3)
Control mature lobes	6	32 ± 1
Control lobes after compensatory growth	5	36 ± 5
Mature lobar transplants	6	32 ± 4
Immature lobar autografts	5	18 ± 1 *
Immature lobar allografts	6	17 ± 3 *

* $p<0.05$ versus first three groups

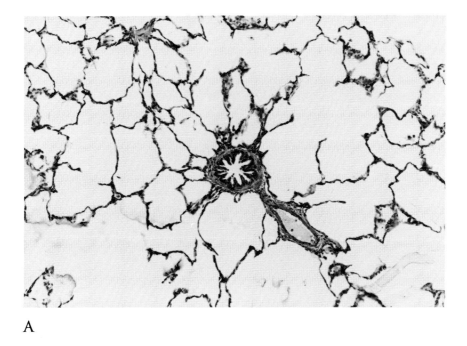

A

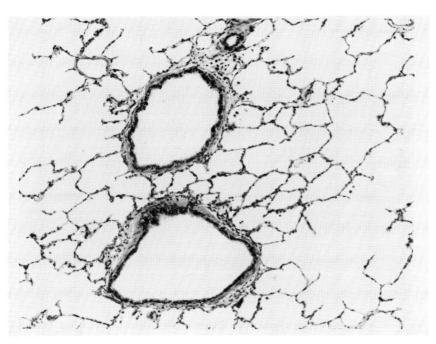

B

Fig. 1. Histologic sections of: A) Transplanted immature whole lung and B) Reduced-size mature lobar transplant. The distal airways of the immature whole lung transplants were consistently smaller than corresponding airways in the reduced-size mature lobar transplants. Pulmonary architecture in both allografts of this porcine model of pediatric lung transplantation was otherwise normal. (H and E stain; 125 x magnification prior to reproduction.)

of postnatal lung development must be completed in the new host in the face of immunosuppressive drugs and potential ongoing rejection. The effects of these insults are unknown. Clinically successful pediatric lung transplantation has not been studied long enough to be able to determine the fate of transplanted immature whole lungs and whether these lungs develop and mature normally. Experimentally, a few studies do exist.

Haverich and his colleagues from Germany were the first to report the growth potential of transplanted immature whole lungs.[9] These investigators used a pig model and transplanted the whole left lung of immature 20 kg pigs. The pigs were allowed to grow while receiving standard immunosuppression and at the end of the growth period underwent analysis of lung growth. The parameters assayed in this study were chest circumference, diameter of the main left lower lobe pulmonary artery and the diameter, length and volume of the main left lower lobe bronchus. The data from this study indicate that the transplanted lungs grew normally when compared to nontransplanted lungs from control animals.[9,10] The diameter of the left lower lobe pulmonary artery was 9.4 ± 0.8 mm in the transplanted lungs and 9.7 ± 1.2 mm in the control lungs. The volume of the left lower lobe bronchus was 2664 ± 266 cubic mm in the transplant lungs and 2499 ± 291 in the control lungs. In addition, pulmonary arteriograms and bronchograms of the transplanted lungs showed no significant narrowing at the anastomoses. While this study clearly demonstrated normal gross development of the transplanted immature lungs, subtle abnormalities of the *distal* airways and pulmonary vascular bed could have gone undetected. Small airway abnormalities are important because it is the smaller, muscular segmental and subsegmental airways that largely determine airway resistance in the absence of obvious anastomotic strictures of the larger airways. Likewise, the distal pulmonary vascular bed is largely responsible for the maintenance of pulmonary artery pressure in response to increases in blood flow through capillary recruitment and vasodilation. In this study, the distal pulmonary vascular bed and bronchial tree were

not evaluated and functional parameters were not reported.

A study which appeared in 1990 examined the growth potential of the transplanted immature rat lung.[8] This was a very elegant study which assessed the lung volume and alveolar number and size of transplanted immature left lungs and the contralateral right lungs six months after transplantation. In this study, the transplanted left lungs were reported to have grown normally as reflected in normal fixed lung volumes and total alveolar number, compared to normal left lungs of control animals.[8] An interesting finding, however, was that the *contralateral right lungs* in the transplanted animals were larger than normal. The investigators concluded that the right lung "appeared not to sense the presence of the transplanted lung, nor was it prevented from growing by the limited amount of space available."[8] While fixed lung volume of the transplanted lungs was normal, functional volume was not assessed and this parameter may have been abnormal. It is known in human children up to the age of five years and possibly even beyond, that loss of functional lung volume results in compensatory growth of the remaining lung tissue so that functioning lung volumes eventually approach normal.[21] In this rat model, whatever the mechanism for stimulating compensatory growth, only the normal right lung was able to respond.[8] Although the transplanted lung grew normally with respect to gross lung volume no *compensatory* growth was seen[8] and functional capacity may have been abnormal, thereby resulting in hypertrophy of the normal right lung.

A study in early 1993 evaluated growth of the transplanted immature primate lung.[11] This study involved the reimplantation of the left lung of eight week old baboons and evaluation of the volume of that lung at 13 weeks and 9 months posttransplant. Reimplantation was done to evaluate only the effects of denervation and not the effects of chronic immunosuppression and rejection. In this study, lung volumes were determined by nitrogen washout and computed tomography (CT).[11] The results showed that the reimplanted left lung volumes increased 91% when measured by nitrogen washout and

75% when measured by CT compared to 85% and 80% for a sham operated animal. In addition, left lung capacity/kilogram body weight was only slightly lower in the reimplanted animals early after transplant compared to age matched controls (20 ± 5 ml/kg vs. 28 ± 3 ml/kg) and was nearly identical to age matched controls by nine months (26 ± 8 ml/kg vs. 24 ± 1 ml/kg).[11] These investigators concluded that in the absence of immunosuppression and rejection, denervation and the insult of transplantation have no long-term deleterious effect on lung volume growth of the immature primate lung.[11]

In a study from our own laboratory which examined long-term airway function and pulmonary mechanics of transplanted immature lungs and reduced-size mature lobes, evaluation was also made of functional lung volume of the transplant by measuring functional residual capacity of the allografts.[7] These results were compared to the volume of nonmanipulated native left lower lobes which were allowed to undergo compensatory growth following left upper lobectomy in early life. Functional residual capacity of the immature whole lungs and reduced-size mature lobar transplants was nearly identical (798 ± 249 ml versus 744 ± 196 ml respectively) and was somewhat smaller than the FRC of left lower lobes which underwent compensatory growth (1135 ± 101 ml), though these differences were not significant.[7] These results indicate an inability of the transplanted lung or lobe, whether immature or mature to undergo *compensatory* growth and were similar to our previous results which showed no increase in FRC of reduced-size mature lobar transplants.[5] Chest radiographs from this study are displayed in Figure 2. The issue of whether or not the immature lung transplants

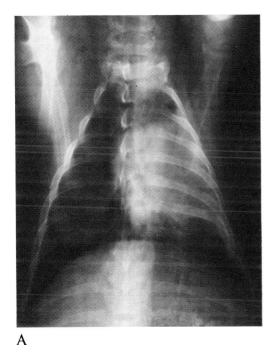

A

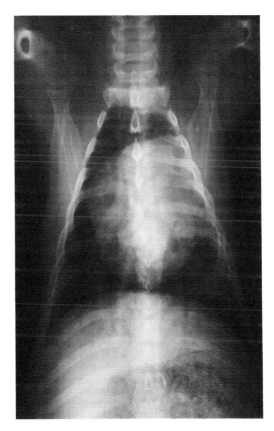

B

Fig. 2. Chest radiographs of: A) transplanted immature whole lung and B) reduced-size mature lobar transplant in a porcine model. Both radiographs taken approximately three months after transplant.

grew normally was not addressed in this particular study.

The studies of growth potential of experimental immature whole lung and reduced-size mature lobar transplants allow us to draw several conclusions:

1. Immature whole lung transplants are capable of some degree of volume growth and alveolar multiplication. The maximum degree of functional volume growth is not known.

2. Immature whole lung transplants display normal growth of the large proximal airways and vessels, however, distal airway growth and development are likely to be abnormal. These subtle abnormalities of development and structural remodeling may only manifest as functional abnormalities.

3. In the presence of a normal contralateral lung, immature whole lung transplants do not display significant *compensatory growth.*

4. Reduced-size lung transplants increase in size following transplantation into a growing recipient, but this is not due to an increase in functional lung volume nor to an increase in number or size of alveoli.

The limitations of studies of growth potential lie in the fact that a normally functioning contralateral lung was always present. It may be that both immature and mature lung tissue, when transplanted into a growing recipient and exposed to various growth factors, could be stimulated into compensatory growth and hypertrophy if appropriate demands were to be placed on it. It is known that in humans and in some experimental animals, when the contralateral pulmonary artery is narrowed or obliterated and the contralateral lung is small, thereby increasing blood flow through the remaining lung, that the remaining normal lung displays an increase in lung volume.[22] The same may be true of *transplanted* lungs. Until long-term survivors of clinical pediatric lung transplantation can be studied, we need to develop a chronic experimental model in which we can preferentially shunt blood to and place a high ventilatory demand on the transplanted lung over time to determine if these are the stimuli needed to cause compensatory growth of the grafted lung. To date such a model has not been developed.

SUMMARY

From the above review of experimental data it would appear that in the setting of a neonate, infant or small child in need of a single lung transplant, a reduced-size mature lobe may be superior to an immature whole lung. At least for the short and medium terms, pulmonary vascular physiology and airway mechanics might be optimal in the reduced-size lobar transplant. In addition, if the reduced-size transplant is harvested from a genetic relative immunologic benefits would likely result. Functional growth of the graft may present a long-term problem, however, and lack of compensatory growth might impact negatively on the long-term functional capacity of the reduced-size transplant. However, the same may hold true for transplanted immature whole lungs. In addition, depending on the reason for which the transplant was done (congenital diaphragmatic hernia with severe pulmonary hypoplasia) there may come a time in the recipient's life when native lung development and function are adequate and the graft could be removed. Or, in cases where continued pulmonary support is needed, the recipient would be old enough to receive a second transplant, either a mature whole lung or a second lobe.

It appears at the present time that both immature whole lung and reduced-size lung transplants hold promise for the young patient with end-stage lung disease in whom no other long-term therapeutic options exist. We need to be open minded and continue to explore all possibilities in order to save these children. Providing them with time through transplantation increases the probability that they will be alive when even greater breakthroughs are made in the field of immunosuppression, immunotolerance or in other means of pulmonary support.

REFERENCES

1. Crombleholme TM, Adzick NS, Longaker MT et al. Reduced-size lung transplantation in neonatal swine: technique and short term physiologic response. Ann Thorac Surg 1990; 49:55-60.

2. McGahren ED, Teague WG, Flanagan TL et al. Airway obstruction after autologous reimplantation of the porcine lobe. J Thorac Cardiovasc Surg 1989; 97(4):587-92.

3. Johnson AM, Teague WG, Flanagan TL, Mcgahren ED, Kron IL. Decreased vascular compliance after reimplantation of the left lower lobe in young pigs. Ann Thorac Surg 1990; 50:277-80.

4. Kern JA, Tribble CG, Chan BBK, Flanagan TL, Kron IL. Reduced-size porcine lung transplantation: long-term studies of pulmonary vascular resistance. Ann Thorac Surg 1992; 53:583-9.

5. Kern JA, Tribble CG, Flanagan TL et al. Growth potential of porcine reduced-size mature pulmonary lobar transplants. J Thorac Cardiovasc Surg 1992; 104:1329-32.

6. Kern JA, Kron IL, Flanagan TL et al. Denervation of the immature porcine lung impairs normal airway development. J Heart Lung Transplant 1993; 12:34-41.

7. Kern JA, Tribble CG, Zografakis JG et al. Analysis of airway function of immature whole lung transplants versus mature lobar transplants. Ann Thorac Surg 1993; In Press.

8. Hislop AA, Odom NJ, McGregor CGA, Haworth SG. Growth potential of the immature transplanted lung. J Thorac Cardiovasc Surg 1990; 100:360-70.

9. Haverich A, Dammenhayn L, Demertzis S, Kemnitz J, Reimers P. Lung growth after experimental pulmonary transplantation. J Heart Lung Transplant 1991; 10:288-95.

10. Dammenhayn L, Haverich A, Demertzis S, Reimers P, Kemnitz J. Growth of lung allografts after experimental transplantation. Thorac Cardiovasc Surg 1991; 39(1):40-3.

11. Thomas DD, Standaert TA, Anton WR et al. Growth potential of he transplanted lung in the infant primate. Ann Thorac Surg 1993; In Press.

12. Rendas A, Branthwaite M, Reid L. Growth of pulmonary circulation in normal pig-structural and cardiopulmonary function. J Appl Physiol 1978; 45:806-17.

13. Allgood RJ, Ebert PA, Sabiston DC. Immediate changes in pulmonary hemodynamics following lung autotransplantation. Ann Surg 1968; 167(3):352-8.

14. Koerner SK, Veith FJ. Hemodynamics of transplanted lungs. Chest 1971; 59(5):531-4.

15. Daicoff GR, Allen PD, Streck CJ. Pulmonary vascular resistance following lung reimplantation and transplantation. Ann Thorc Surg 1970; 9(6):569-79.

16. Veith FJ, Montefusco CM. Long-term fate of autografts charged with providing total pulmonary function. Ann Surg 1979; 190(5):654-6.

17. Veith FJ, Richards L. Lung transplantation with simultaneous contralateral pulmonary artery ligation. Surg Gynecol Obstet 1969; 129:768-74.

18. Wain JC, Suen HC, Donahue DM, Ryan DP. Lobar lung allografts: acute studies with an elevated native pulmonary vascular resistance. Surg Forum 1991; XLII:415-7.

19. Hislop AA, Wigglesworth JS, Desai R. Alveolar development in the human fetus and infant. Early human development 1986; 13:1-11.

20. Hobson CE, Teague WG, Tribble CG et al. Denervation of transplanted porcine lung causes airway obstruction. Ann Thorac Surg 1991; 52:1295-9.

21. Laros CD, Westermann CJJ. Dilatation, compensatory growth, or both after pneumonectomy during childhood and adolescence. J Thorac Cardiovasc Surg 1987; 93:570-6.

22. Tartter P, Goss R. Compensatory pulmonary hypertrophy after incapacitation of one lung in the rat. J Thorac Cardiovasc Surg 1973; 66:147-52.

CHAPTER 7

REDUCED-SIZE LUNG TRANSPLANTATION: CLINICAL EXPERIENCE

Pierre R. Theodore
Vaughn A. Starnes

INTRODUCTION

Since Hardy's first efforts at clinical lung transplantation, several modifica tions of surgical technique and perioperative care have been addressed.[1] The introduction of cyclosporine and other successful immunosuppressive agents has greatly improved the success rates of solid organ transplantation. Advances in the standards of intensive care management, technical refinements of the operations and a better understanding of the immunology and diagnosis of rejection have contributed to the expanding clinical applicability of lung transplantation.

Among the issues related to transplantation that have proved most resistant to solution are donor shortages and chronic rejection. Particularly in the pediatric population, a shortage of donor organs has severely limited the applicability of more widespread lung transplantation. To address the issues of donor organ shortage and optimal tissue matching, both cadaveric and living related lobar transplants have been performed. To date, unilateral and bilateral lobar transplantations have resulted in satisfactory intermediate survival. Initial outcomes have been encouraging suggesting that lobar transplantation may become a more widely used therapeutic option in the management of end-stage pulmonary

Reduced-size Lung Transplantation, edited by John A. Kern, M.D. and Irving L. Kron, M.D.; © 1993 R.G. Landes Company.

disease in children and in some adults. In the setting of the decompensating or end-stage patient, living related reduced-size lung transplantation can provide a donor source within the limited time constraints of these frequently urgent clinical situations.

INDICATIONS FOR LOBAR TRANSPLANTATION

The indications for lobar transplantation generally do not differ from those for whole lung transplantation. All patients were listed for conventional transplantation, but each experienced acute decompensations requiring assessment for lobar transplantation. At the time of transplantation all patients were oxygen dependent. Cyanosis, increased supplemental oxygen demands and progressive right heart failure were the primary indications for consideration for urgent transplantation.

Patients with end-stage disease of either restrictive or obstructive type are considered for transplantation. It has been our opinion that single lung transplantation is best suited to restrictive lung diseases. However, in contrast to the adult population isolated pulmonary fibrosis is an uncommon cause of end-stage lung disease in pediatric patients. Additionally, patients with severe pulmonary vascular disease, either primary or in association with cardiac defects, are evaluated for transplantation. The diagnoses for patients undergoing lobar transplantation are summarized in Table 1.

In the setting of a neonate with severe pulmonary hypoplasia associated with congenital diaphragmatic hernia, lobar transplantation can represent an option of preference. The size requirements for these youngest of patients often precludes the use of a cadaveric size-matched whole lung. For this population the shortage of neonatal donors without lung disease is profound and the urgency of the clinical scenario may not allow for a lengthy wait for a satisfactory cadaveric whole immature lung.

Lobar transplantation has been performed in patients with both primary pulmonary hypertension and Eisenmenger's syndrome. Primary pulmonary hypertension within the pediatric population is a less common indication for single lung (or lobar) transplantation than pulmonary hypertension associated with an uncorrected congenital cardiac lesion. For Eisenmenger's syndrome patients failure of palliative surgery for the management of elevated pulmonary artery pressures and progressive decline in clinical status are potential indications for lobar transplantation with correction of the cardiac defect at the time of operation.

Cystic fibrosis (CF) provides certain challenges to the surgeon that cannot be met with the transplantation of a single lung. Though CF is a systemic disease, bronchopulmonary disease is the most prominent cause of mortality in this patient population. Our one patient chosen

---

Table 1. *Primary Diagnoses of Patients Undergoing Lobar Transplantation*

Fibrotic Disease
   Bronchopulmonary Dysplasia
   Cystic Fibrosis

Pulmonary Vascular Disease
   Eisenmenger's Syndrome
   Primary Pulmonary Hypertension
   Inadequate pulmonary vasculature development in association with
      congenital diaphragmatic hernia.

---

for bilateral lobar transplantation had been managed successfully medically into young adulthood. However, transplantation was considered as her rapidly progressing pulmonary disease, inadequate nutrition and oxygen dependence became increasingly resistant to nonsurgical management. The near universal colonization of the lung with Aspergillus species and mixed bacterial flora prevents the preservation of a native lung and is an indication for bilateral lung replacement in CF patients reaching end stage. Specific indications for lung transplantation in CF patients include pulmonary function test indicating FEV_1 less than 25–30% of predicted value.[2]

We presently do not consider for transplantation patients with brittle diabetes mellitus, collagen vascular disease or colonization with resistant organisms. Patients with poor renal or hepatic function are generally not transplanted in our program. Silent hepatic dysfunction associated with primary pulmonary hypertension is common and is associated with the passive congestion resulting from a failing right ventricle. Total bilirubin should be below 2.5 mg/dl in older children or young adults being considered for lobar transplantation.[3] Transplantation is contraindicated in CF patients with recurrent or active pancreatitis. We have relaxed our initial requirements that patients be completely weaned from steroids at the time of surgery. However, individuals on systemic steroids for their underlying lung disease should be weaned to alternate day dosing with a maximum dose of less than 20 mg of prednisone on alternate days.

PREOPERATIVE ASSESSMENTS

DONOR EVALUATION

Donor selection in the case of living related lung transplantation involves assessment of both physiologic and psychosocial factors (Table 2). As with all transplants involving pediatric patients the presence of a stable supportive environment prepared for the long-term management of the recipient must be assured. The evaluation of both recipient and donors in consultation with social workers and a psychiatric team is required to fully assess patient coping skills and psychosocial stability. It is of utmost importance that the recipients have an intact support system and that parents and patients are committed to the task of long-term management.

Potential donors are ABO and tissue typed for assessment of the optimal donor. We do not consider HLA type mismatching a contraindication to reduced-size lung transplantation despite recent clinical data indicating that HLA tissue typing contributes to improved long-term survival of pulmonary allografts. Tissue matching appears to be most critical at the DR locus of the MHC II gene.[4] Our longest surviving patient is only two years from transplantation and hence convincing data documenting the immunologic advantage of living related lung transplantation are

---

Table 2. Donor Selection Criteria for Living Related Lung Transplantation

ABO match
Normal Chest X-ray
Normal spirometry and normal arterial blood gas values
Psychosocially intact
Negative smoking history (preferable)
No transmittable infection

pending. Chest radiographs, spirometry, FEV_1, bronchoscopy, ventilation perfusion (V/Q) scanning and cardiac evaluation represent the cornerstones of the living related donor evaluation. Additionally, details of the medical history such as smoking, persistent upper respiratory tract infection, chest trauma or transmittable disease must be considered. Of our living related donors only one had a notable smoking history. Although donor smoking history is a relative contraindication, the severity of the clinical scenario may warrant the use of the lobe of an asymptomatic smoker.

RECIPIENT ASSESSMENT

The recipient preoperative evaluation consists of baseline pulmonary function testing including FEV25-75, FRC and TLC (Table 3). Additionally, the recipient upper respiratory tract should be cultured for the presence of bacterial colonization. Given the compromised immune system of the transplant recipient it is desirable to manage any prominent nidus of infection in the preoperative period. Additionally, the CMV status of the recipient is determined. We routinely place patients receiving grafts from CMV antibody positive donors on prophylactic ganciclovir postoperatively. Patients with a history of blood transfusion, previous operation or pregnancy are screened for preformed cytoreactive antibodies to donor antigens.

The importance of a thorough cardiac evaluation warrants mentioning. Patients with mild to moderate right ventricular dysfunction frequently show a return toward normal cardiac function with single lobe transplantation due to the decrease in right ventricular afterload. The implantation of lung tissue with normal vascular compliance results in relief of right ventricular strain.[5,6] Patients with severe cardiac dysfunction, e.g. evidence of biventricular failure, are not likely to demonstrate improvement of cardiac indices with single lung transplantation. We consider right ventricular ejection fractions greater than 15–20% sufficient evidence of "reversible ventricular dysfunction". However, patients with significant left heart dysfunction (LVEF< 35%, LVEDP>12 mm Hg) are likely to be better candidates for heart-lung transplantation.

SURGICAL TECHNIQUE

Cardiopulmonary bypass has been required for all patients. We have utilized bicaval-aorto bypass. The diminutive femoral vessels may not be sufficient for femoral artery-femoral vein bypass in smaller patients. Though some investigators have employed a low flow partial bypass for single lung patients with primary pulmonary hypertension, our preference has been full bypass for those patients undergoing lobar transplantation.[7] One patient was operated on while remaining on an ECMO circuit. In several of our whole lung transplantations and in our bilateral lobar transplantation we have utilized an in line leukocyte filter.

Table 3. Inpatient Evaluation for Recipient

ABO typing
Pulmonary Function Tests, V/Q scan, Chest radiography
Cardiac evaluation
Psychosocial evaluation
Laboratory work up (ABG, CBC, Electrolytes, BUN, Cr, Liver Function Tests)

Monitoring includes the placement of a pulmonary artery catheter opposite the side to be transplanted, pulse oximetry, central venous pressure and arterial pressure. Additionally, sophisticated ventilation techniques should be available including high frequency ventilation and differential ventilation of the native and grafted lungs.

DONOR OPERATION

The donor lobe is approached through a posterolateral thoracotomy. For our single lobe transplantations we have employed a standard posterolateral approach at the level of the 6th intercostal space for lower lobes (4th intercostal space for upper lobes). The lobes are isolated via blunt and sharp dissection with an attempt to attain satisfactory pulmonary artery length. Once the fissures are satisfactorily developed the donor is heparinized. Laboratory experience has demonstrated that early heparinization significantly complicates the lobectomy particularly when the fissures are poorly developed. For right upper lobectomy an attempt is made to isolate all of the arteries going to the lobe. We remove the right upper lobe arteries as a Carrel patch with reconstruction using pericardium if needed.

PRESERVATION AND MANAGEMENT OF THE LOBE

At a sterile back table the donor lobe bronchus is intubated with a #6 uncuffed tube and the lobe is hand ventilated at rate of 10 "breaths" per minute of room air. Using a 14 F catheter the lobar artery is cannulated and the orifice is cinched shut with umbilical tape. The lobar pulmonary artery is infused with a 4°C modified Euro-Collins solution with PGE_1 added in an initial bolus. Upon completion of pulmonoplegia with adequate blanching of the entire parenchyma and clear effluent from the pulmonary vein the lobe is carefully given a final large breath with attention to all sites of atelectasis, the lobar bronchus is clamped and the lobe is transported

for implantation immersed in cold physiologic solution (Fig. 1). Cadaveric donor procedures differ in that we prefer to remove the heart and lungs en bloc and continue the dissection of the lobe at a sterile back table.

RECIPIENT OPERATION

Single lobe recipients are approached through a posterolateral thoracotomy. In the case of our CF patient, a transverse thoracosternotomy incision was employed (clam shell incision) which readily provides sufficient bilateral exposure for the institution of bicaval cardiopulmonary bypass. In CF patients, significant bleeding complications are frequently associated with difficult to reach areas of the thorax (apices, directly posterior to the hilum). We have found that the clam shell incision allows for improved access to these problematic regions. For those patients that are likely to have significant pleural adhesions (previous thoracotomy, CF, and pleurodesis) the clam shell incision is the preferred approach.

Donor and recipient operations are coordinated to minimize the ischemic time of the graft. With appropriate timing the recipient's hilar structures are isolated. Following arrival of the graft the recipient pneumonectomy is completed using vascular staples on the pulmonary veins and arteries and TA 30 staples on the mainstem bronchus. The pulmonary artery is divided as distal as is technically feasible with the excess trimmed at the time of implantation of the reduced-size lobe. The veins are divided at the hilum in order to provide adequate length for the venous anastomosis.

The bronchus is anastomosed first as described by Trinkle with a posterior row of running proline suture and an anterior row of horizontal mattress sutures.[8] Limiting the amount of peribronchial dissection and mild telescoping of donor into recipient bronchus has provided excellent healing of the airway anastomosis without the need for omental wraps. We routinely mobilize a pedicle of pericardium to provide some protection for the bronchial

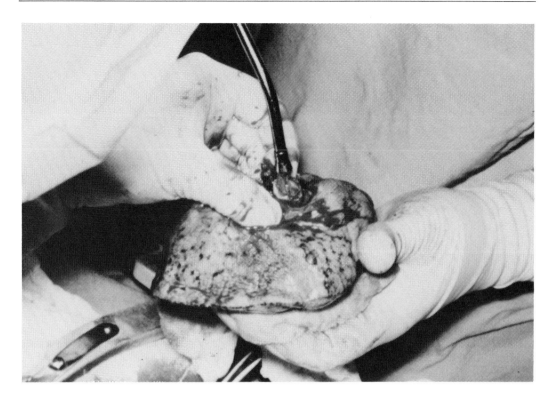

Fig. 1. Donor left lower lobe immediately after harvesting from living related donor.

anastomosis. The venous anastomosis is performed in a running fashion with the lobar vein of the donor anastomosed to the *superior pulmonary vein* of the recipient. The anastomosis of the bronchus brings the donor lobar vein in closest approximation to the superior pulmonary vein of the recipient. We have not found the use of left atrial cuffs beneficial in lobar transplantation, though use of a cuff may be indicated in the event that vein-to-vein anastomosis is not technically feasible. The arterial anastomosis is completed using 5-0 proline suture. We allow the pulmonary vasculature to de-air by leaving the venous anastomosis untied until venting of air has occurred following unclamping of the pulmonary artery. After re-perfusion of the reduced-size lobe and weaning from cardiopulmonary bypass, the recipient is pulsed with 10–15 mg/kg of methylprednisolone IV. The chest is closed in layers and two right angled thoracic catheters are left in place. Immediately following the operation the patient is bronchoscoped for signs of technical complications.

RESULTS OF CLINICAL REDUCED-SIZE LUNG TRANSPLANTATION

Our experience consists of reduced-size lobar transplantation in five patients varying in age from 17 days to 21 years as summarized in Table 4. Four of the patients received single lobes and our only adult patient was the recipient of bilateral living related reduced-size lung transplants with both mother and father serving as donors (Fig. 2).

Of the five patients who have undergone lobar transplantation, there was one early mortality. Of the remaining four recipients three have attained normal activity without the need for supplemental oxygen. The one

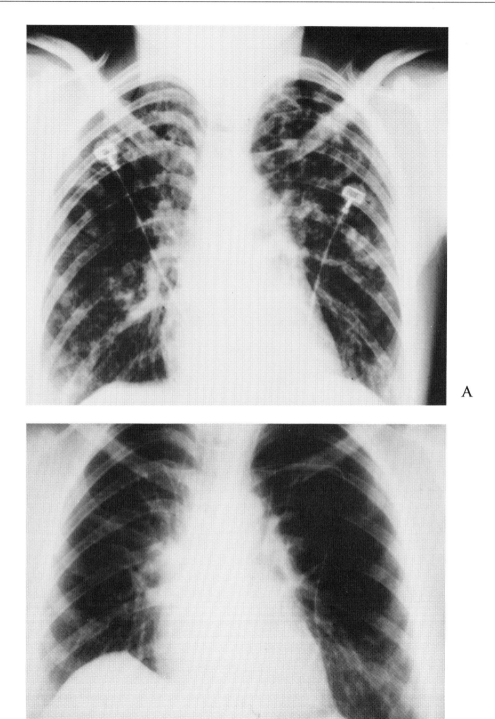

Fig. 2. Pre-(A) and post-(B) operative chest radiographs of patient with cystic fibrosis. This patient received bilateral living related reduced-size lobar transplants.

mortality involved a patient that developed severe reperfusion pulmonary edema and died due to respiratory failure immediately following surgery. Our surgical technique did not involve the use of an omental wrap nor bronchial artery revascularization. No airway complications were encountered.

No cases of obliterative bronchiolitis (OB) have yet been seen. In earlier series we have found the incidence of OB to be as high as 35% in long-term single lung transplants. In spite of the fact that we have not seen any cases of OB in these intermediate term lobar transplant recipients, greater long-term experience is likely to yield this classic pattern of chronic rejection. No CMV infections have complicated the postoperative courses of the recipients.

With respect to complications involving the donors, a prolonged air leak was encountered in one living related lobar donor (18 days). No donor has had long-term compromise of respiratory function as a result of lobectomy.

Episodes of acute rejection as diagnosed by chest radiography, clinical findings and transbronchial biopsy (TBB) have been minimal in the neonate transplanted with a cadaveric lobe for pulmonary hypoplasia associated with diaphragmatic hernia and in the one adult patient with bilateral living related lobar transplants. These two patients experienced mild early rejection but have been free of rejection since discharged from the hospital. One patient encountered significant rejection complications as a result of medical noncompliance and is presently at home on supplemental oxygen therapy.

The reduced-size grafts received most of the pulmonary artery blood flow as documented by perfusion scanning (Table 4). These patients had marked elevations of pulmonary vascular resistance in the native lung. As a consequence of the increased vascular resistance, prominent shunting to the compliant vascular bed of the transplanted lobe occurred. The degree of shunting into the transplanted lobe ranged from 74% to 99% to the reduced-size grafts. In our one case of bilateral lobar transplantation pulmonary blood flow was nearly evenly distributed to both sides (52% and 48%).

IMMUNOSUPPRESSION AND REJECTION MANAGEMENT

The issue of perioperative steroid use in the management of the lung transplant recipient has been strongly debated. In spite of early reports that use of steroids was a cause of complications of the airway

Table 4. Recipients of Reduced-size Lung Transplantation

AGE	DX	LOBE	DONOR	OUTCOME	SCAN
21 yrs	CF	RLL/LLL (Bilateral)	LR-Mother (49) LR-Father (55)	Lived	52% 48%
12 yrs	BPD	RUL	LR-Mother (44)	Lived	74%
4 yrs	ES	RML	LR-Father (33)	Died	
28 days	PPH	LUL	CAD (2 yrs)	Lived	99%
17 days	DH	RUL/RML	CAD (6 mo)	Lived	85%

CF-Cystic Fibrosis, BPD-Bronchopulmonary Dysplasia, PPH-Primary Pulmonary Hypertension, ES-Eisenmenger's Syndrome, DH-Diaphragmatic Hernia, Scan-Ventilation/Perfusion Scan, LR-Living related, CAD-Cadaveric Donor

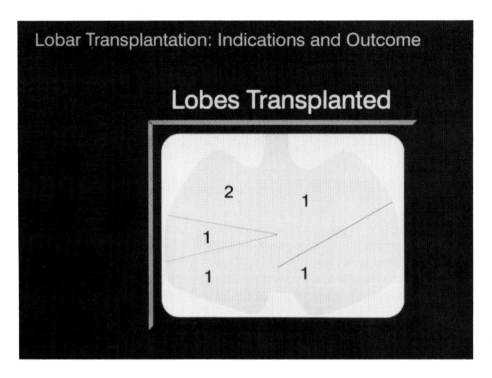

Fig. 3. Pulmonary lobes used for reduced-size lung transplants to date.

anastomosis, present practice suggests that the judicious use of steroids in the immediate postoperative period is not associated with dehiscence of the bronchial anastomosis or stricture formation. Many investigators routinely employ the use of steroids in the early postoperative period.[9] Nevertheless, we try to avoid the use of steroids for the first week posttransplantation.[10] Cyclosporine is started preoperatively in patients undergoing living related lobar transplantation. Immunosuppression in all patients is induced via the use of the polyclonal antibody anti-thymocyte globulin (10–15mg/kg) and cyclosporine A at a dose of 1–2 mg/kg/day IV to a serum level of 150–250 ng/ml. Additionally, azathioprine is given to leukocyte tolerance (4000 cells/ml). As soon as oral medications are tolerated, the cyclosporine (7–12mg/kg) and azathioprine (1–2 mg/kg) are switched to oral preparations and given in two (divided) daily doses. Beyond one week postoperatively, daily doses of steroids (0.6 mg/kg PO) are

administered. Over the course of one month the recipient is gradually tapered to 0.2 mg/kg of prednisone.

We have treated reduced-size lung rejection episodes with a three-day course of methylprednisolone in a (15 mg/kg/day). Generally, the response to methylprednisolone is excellent with an improvement in clinical status of the patient within 24 hours. In the event a rejection episode does not respond to pulse steroids, the monoclonal antibody OKT3 (0.1–0.2 mg/kg up to a maximum of 5 mg/day) has been our standard second line of therapy. However, patients not responding to initial boluses of methylprednisolone should be re-evaluated for the presence of infection, as rejection and infection are by no means mutually exclusive phenomena.

WHICH LOBE TO TRANSPLANT

The lobe chosen to transplant is a source of debate and a topic of our experimental investigations. We have attempted transplantation of all lobes (Fig. 3). From the standpoint of technical feasibility the left lower lobe is readily accessed and the pulmonary vessels and lobar bronchi form a triad allowing for relatively straightforward anastomoses during implantation without the need for reconstruction using pericardium or homograft. The right upper lobe is also suitable for transplantation. However, the multiple lobar arteries which are removed as a Carrel patch and reconstructed with pericardium complicates the use of this lobe. We have had success with this strategy in the harvest of the right upper lobe and angiographic confirmation suggests that perfusion has not been compromised by this approach. The right middle lobe has proved to be easily accessed, but it has been suggested that the right middle lobe may not have a sufficiently developed microvascular bed.[11] Resection of the right lower lobe can result in compromise of the right middle lobe bronchus given its proximity to the right lower lobe bronchus.

In part, the lobe selected for transplantation is a function of the individual anatomy of the donor in addition to the previous surgical history. Donors with near complete fissuring may present several lobes that are resectable for transplantation. To the contrary, donors with incomplete fissuring require more sharp dissection and the application of surgical staplers to complete the fissure. It has been our preference to limit sharp dissection and stapling to the greatest degree possible.

From a physiologic standpoint, it is not clear which of the lobes is best capable of handling the demands of the significant shunting of cardiac output that occurs through the graft posttransplantation. However, the right middle lobe is thought to be, physiologically, a segment with a relatively deficient ratio of vascular surface to parenchymal lung displacement. Although considerable more investigation into the issue of differential lobar vascular physiology remains to be done, we presently do not consider the right middle lobe ideal for reduced-size lung transplantation.

We have had problems with the use of lung tissue in which the disparity in donor to recipient body weight approached 6 to 1 (Table 5). In such cases, pruning the periphery of the lobe for the size constraints of the recipient thorax may result in significant loss of the microvascular bed. In the event of extreme size mismatches "shoe horning" of the lobe and excessive pruning of the distal parenchyma have the similar effect of compromising the microvascular blood flow, potentially leading to transudation of fluid and poor ventilation, particularly in the setting of the interruption of lymphatic flow associated with transplantation. In our one early mortality, significant pulmonary edema developed secondary to the excessive blood flow through a transplanted right middle lobe with an apparent inadequate microvascular bed. This was partially confirmed by the lack of pulmonary pressure drop following release of the pulmonary artery clamp.

Obtaining a good match of recipient thoracic volume to lobar volume is the most important concern when choosing a mature lobe for transplantation. Proper assessment of the thoracic dimensions of the recipient and estimation of the volume of the lobe to be implanted are critical preoperative parameters of reduced-size lobar transplantation. Full spirometry and V/Q scanning with segmental percentages of the upper, middle and lower zones permit adequate approximation of the FEV_1 and FVC of potential donor lobes. Additionally, computerized tomographic evaluation of lung volume allows for estimation of donor lobar volumes which bears heavily on the choice of lobe(s) for transplantation. By these measures the lobe chosen can be best matched with the physiologic needs of the recipient. Generally, the lower lobes are preferable given the technical accessibility and their prominent vasculature.

COMMENTS

Transbronchial biopsy (TBB) is our standard in the diagnosis of rejection for patients in whom biopsy is technically feasible.

Recipients are biopsied one week following transplantation and upon any signs of clinical deterioration. The use of open lung biopsy in this limited series of patients has not been required. Serial pulmonary function testing has been demonstrated to be a useful adjunct to TBB in the early diagnosis of rejection, with the FEV25-75 level being most closely correlated with rejection.[12] Simple PFTs (FEV_1 and VC) have the advantage of being monitored in the home and may provide some means of early detection of decline in respiratory function.[13]

The Achilles heel of bilateral living related lobar transplantation is the need for two compatible donors and the resources to coordinate three separate operations. The role of reduced-size lobar transplantation for cystic fibrosis is yet to be defined. For larger patients who have been successfully managed medically into adulthood, lobar transplantation may not provide sufficient lung tissue for the older patient's needs. Thus, reduced-size lobar transplantation is not likely to entirely supplant bilateral lung transplantation or heart-lung domino procedures in adult CF patients with end-stage lung disease. As a consequence of the lack of an available double lung donor for a rapidly decompensating patient, however, our one adult CF patient underwent lobar transplantation receiving the right lower lobe of the mother and the left lower lobe of the father with excellent intermediate term outcome.

Patients with secondary pulmonary hypertension (Eisenmenger's syndrome), primary pulmonary hypertension or certain parenchymal diseases, i.e. bronchopulmonary dysplasia, can be expected to shunt the majority of cardiac output through the transplanted lobe. Careful selection of donor tissue must take this posttransplant shunt phenomenon into consideration. The lobe or lobes chosen for transplantation must be capable of handling the majority of the cardiac output which may exclude some lobes from consideration, i.e. the right middle lobe.

The pediatric patient with cardiopulmonary disease is a challenge to manage successfully.

Improvements in intensive care and surgical techniques have resulted in growing applications of transplantation in the pediatric population. Our present experience with clinical lobar transplantation suggests that living related reduced-size transplantation may be a viable therapeutic option for certain patients with severe end-stage lung disease. The profound shortage of donor organs remains a principle factor limiting the growth of pulmonary transplant programs.[14] This shortage is most significant within the pediatric population where lungs suitable for transplantation remain exceedingly rare. The use of ECMO as a bridge to transplantation has met with some success, however, this strategy does not function to alleviate donor shortage. In some cases, the use of a reduced-size lobar allograft may serve as "in vivo ECMO" support while the native lung develops the capacity to function adequately. Improvements in the management of donors and the coordination of transplant efforts are likely to contribute to the solution of the donor shortage in the adult population, but it is not clear that such efforts will have much effect in improving the shortage for younger patients. Lobar transplantation has been developed to respond in part to the particular shortage of satisfactory immature whole lung donors.

The potential immunologic advantages of living related lobar transplantation are also attractive. The matching of lung tissue is not yet a reality in cadaveric donors given the ischemic time constraints for lung allografts. Proper tissue matching may allow for improved long-term graft function and reduced incidence of chronic rejection. Greater experience will determine the validity of this theoretical advantage.

FUTURE DIRECTIONS

In spite of the promising initial experience with reduced-size lung transplantation, several critical issues need to be investigated further. The capacity of mature lobes to develop in proportion with the increasing demands of the growing child is unclear. A fair amount of experimental data indicate that *immature* lungs retain some ability to develop after transplantation but the long-term changes in mature lobes used for transplantation have not been fully determined.[15,16] It appears that the transplanted immature lung has some ability to compensate for the demands of the growing patient. This capacity may not be limited to immature lungs. It is essential to clinically examine the mature lobe's ability to either develop new gas exchanging units or hyperinflate without the destructive changes of emphysema. Additionally the causes and mechanisms of pulmonary hypertension are yet to be fully elucidated. The wide scale application of this novel therapeutic modality depends in large part on the answers to these and similar questions. However, despite the significant amount of investigation that remains to be done regarding reduced-size lung transplantation, this novel approach represents a viable therapeutic option for young patients with end-stage pulmonary disease.

REFERENCES

1. Hardy JD, Webb WR, Dalton ML, Walker GR. Lung homotransplantation in humans. JAMA 1963; 186:1065-74.
2. Marshall SE, Kramer MK, Lewiston NJ, Starnes VA, Theodore J. Selection and evaluation of recipients for heart-lung and lung transplantation. Chest 1990; 98:1488-94.
3. Starnes VA. Heart lung transplantation; indications, technique and result. Chest Surg Clin North America 1993:pp.113-21.
4. Iwaki Y, Yoshida Y, Griffith B. HLA matching effect in lung transplantation. In press.
5. Starnes VA, Stinson EB, Oyer PE, Theodore J, Kramer MR, Marshall S, Shumway NE. Single lung transplantation: a new therapeutic option for patients with pulmonary hypertension. Transplant Proc 1991; 23:1209-10.
6. Waters P. Single lung transplantation: indications and technique. Semin Thorac Cardiovasc Surg 1992; 4:90-4.
7. Cooper J. The current status of lung transplantation. Archives of Surgery. In: Advances in Surgery 1992; 25:259-307.
8. Calhoon JH, Pearson FG, Patterson GA et al. Technique of successful lung transplantation in humans. J Thorac Cardiovasc Surg 1987; 93:173-81.
9. Shumway SJ. Rejection and immunosuppression in lung transplantation. Clin Chest Surg 1993; 3:145-55.
10. Starnes VA, Oyer PE, Bernstein D, Baum D, Gamberg P, Miller J, Shumway NE. Heart, heart-lung and lung transplantation in the first year of life. Ann Thorac Surg 1992; te:306-10.
11. Starnes VA, Lewiston NJ, Luikart H et al. Current trends in lung transplantation. J Thorac Cardiovasc Surg 1992; 104:1060-6.
12. Kirby TJ, Mehta A, Rice TW, Gephardt GN. Diagnosis and management of acute and chronic rejection. Semin Thorac Cardiovasc Surg 1992; 4:126-31.
13. Otulana BA, Higenbottam TW, Hutter J et al. Close pulmonary monitoring of lung function in heart-lung transplants allows early detection of pulmonary rejection and infection. Am Rev Respir Dis 1988; 137:245-52.
14. Hakim M, Higenbottam T, Bethune D et al. Selection and procurement of combined heart and lung grafts for transplantation. J Thorac Cardiovasc Surg 1988; 95:474-8.
15. Hislop AA, Odom NJ, McGregor GC et al. Growth potential of the immature transplanted lung. J Thorac Cardiovasc Surg 1990; 100:360-70.
16. Haverich A, Dammenhayn L, Demertizis J et al. Lung growth after experimental lung transplantation. J Heart Lung Transplant 1991; 10:288-95.

CHAPTER 8

ETHICAL CONSIDERATIONS IN LIVE DONOR LUNG TRANSPLANTATION

Douglas K. Martin
Peter A. Singer
Mark Siegler

INTRODUCTION

Only recently has lung transplantation gained acceptance as a safe and effective treatment option for patients suffering from end-stage pulmonary disease.[1] Between 1963 and 1980 38 lung transplants were attempted with little success.[2] In the past decade, however, the introduction of cyclosporine along with improved surgical techniques, have resulted in one-year survival rates of 71%, and this has encouraged more patients to choose lung transplantation. Unfortunately, the number of cadaveric lungs donated for transplant is not keeping pace with the demand. Four hundred single lung transplants were performed in the U.S. in 1991, twice as many as in 1990.[3] Nevertheless, in September 1992 there were 937 people on the UNOS waiting list for a new lung,[4] up from 677 in December 1991[5] and 309 in December 1990.[6] As a result, many patients accepted for lung transplantation programs die while awaiting a suitable donor; there were 54 such deaths in the U.S. in 1990.[7] Transplanting lungs from live donors may help to reduce this shortage and save lives; it may also decrease pretransplant morbidity.

To date, live donor lung transplantation (LDLT) has been attempted in five patients, ages 4, 5, 9, and 12,[8] and a 22 year old woman with cystic fibrosis. Regarding the four children, two died in the operating room, one is alive but her graft degenerated due to noncompliance and had to be removed, and the fourth child is alive but repeated viral infections have impaired her respiratory function

Reduced-size Lung Transplantation, edited by John A. Kern, M.D. and Irving L. Kron, M.D.; © 1993 R.G. Landes Company.

to the level she had prior to transplant. The operation on the 22 year old woman took place on January 29, 1993 in Los Angeles, and was unusual in that each of the recipient's parents donated a lung segment (as reported in the *Chicago Tribune,* January 30, 1993, in Section I, page 4).

LDLT has raised ethical questions. For example, a *New York Times* headline reporting on one of the five recipients read: "Lungs from parents fail to save girl, 9, and doctors assess ethics."[9] The purpose of this chapter is to evaluate the ethical issues related to LDLT. Before focusing specifically on LDLT, we begin with a description of the conceptual framework of research ethics.

PRINCIPLES OF RESEARCH ETHICS

Sometimes the most difficult part of research ethics is deciding whether a procedure is research as opposed to clinical practice. Levine has provided a way of making this distinction.[10] A procedure which uses a previously validated means and which is intended solely for the benefit of the patient is known as 'treatment' or 'practice'. The goal of practice is diagnosis, prevention or therapy. Even standard clinical practices do not guarantee a good outcome, but the uncertainty of outcome is common to both clinical and research interventions. A procedure which uses a novel or unproven means and which is intended solely for the benefit of the patient is called 'innovative treatment' or 'nonvalidated practice'. Although generalizable medical knowledge may be derived from the procedure, this is not the primary intent. A procedure, validated or not, which is intended both to benefit the patient and to provide generalizable knowledge is known as 'research'. Lastly, a procedure intended solely to provide generalizable knowledge is called 'practice for the benefit of others'. (Levine has argued against using the terms 'therapeutic' and 'nontherapeutic' research, stating that the distinction between the terms is illogical.[10,11]

LDLT is innovative and has no proven efficacy. Therefore, we believe that LDLT,

which is intended primarily for the benefit of the recipient, is innovative treatment. However, the distinction between innovative treatment and research is a fine one. For instance, the guidelines of the Medical Research Council of Canada state that innovative transplant therapy should be regarded as research.[12] Thus, we recommend that this innovative procedure be undertaken within a peer reviewed research protocol. This would ensure that the medical knowledge gleaned from the procedure will provide maximum benefit to future patients. In either case, the conceptual framework which guides our ethical analysis will be that of research ethics.[13]

Research ethics of the modern era was shaped by the Nuremberg Code which was a response to the atrocities committed by Nazi doctors on unconsenting war prisoners. The Nuremberg Code emphasized the moral obligation of the researcher to obtain the voluntary informed consent of every subject involved in any medical research.[14] Furthermore, it stated that research with human subjects could only be morally justified when the benefits to society (or the "humanitarian importance") exceeded the degree of risk. Thus, informed consent and a favorable risk/benefit analysis became the bedrock of all future analyses of research ethics.

The World Medical Association's Declaration of Helsinki, currently in its fourth version,[15] further entrenched informed consent and a favorable risk/benefit analysis as the major ethical standards for biomedical research with human subjects. However, in the Declaration of Helsinki the concept of benefit was refocussed such that "medical research is (only) justified by its potential diagnostic or therapeutic value to the patient." Other organizations which have published research ethics guidelines, for example the Council for International Organizations of Medical Sciences[16] (CIOMS) and the Medical Research Council of Canada[12] (MRC), have reinforced these moral requirements.

In the U.S., The Belmont Report: Ethical Principles and Guidelines for the Protection of Human Subjects of Research[17] described three ethical principles which are particularly relevant to research involving human subjects: respect for persons, beneficence, and justice. The application of these ethical principles is relevant to analyzing the practical issues of consent, potential harms and benefits, and an additional consideration, subject selection. Since the publication of the Belmont report in 1979 the Department of Health and Human Services Regulations has included a favorable risk/benefit proportion, voluntary informed consent, and an equitable selection of subjects as legal requirements for any federally funded research involving human subjects.[18]

We will examine these three ethical requirements in the context of LDLT and outline steps which will help to ensure the ethical acceptability of the research. Also, since LDLT involves at least two patients — one or two donors and a recipient—both recipient and donor perspectives will be considered in our analysis. Furthermore, both substantive and procedural issues (such as the role of the Institutional Review Board) will be considered. Experience with the development of live donor liver transplantation has demonstrated the potential usefulness of a comprehensive analysis of the ethical issues before undertaking such innovative procedures.[19–21] We have also previously published such an analysis of LDLT.[22] The purpose of this chapter is to analyze the ethical issues in LDLT prospectively, that is, before the procedure becomes widely available. Our goal in doing this is to encourage surgeons, patients, institutions and the public to consider the ethical issues involved in this innovate procedure and to address areas of disagreement before LDLT becomes widely disseminated.

POTENTIAL HARMS AND BENEFITS

In U.S. legislation[23] and other guidelines[12,16,24] research is deemed ethically acceptable when risks to subjects are reasonable in relation to, or are outweighed by, the potential benefits to subjects. Moreover, the ethical principle of beneficence obliges clinical investigators and members of their institutions to take steps to maximize benefits and minimize harms to subjects of research. Since LDLT involves potential risk to a healthy volunteer, this obligation is the dominant ethical issue. In this section we will describe the potential harms and benefits of LDLT as well as its potential impact on the health care system. In subsequent sections we address the difficulty of weighing the harms and benefits of LDLT.

RECIPIENTS

Harms

Because of the paucity of experience with LDLT, specifying the extent and probability of harm is difficult. The risks to recipients of cadaveric single lung transplants[25] will at least help in predicting the risks of LDLT. (Of course, the relevant consideration here is the incremental risk to the recipient of receiving a lung segment from a live donor compared to a cadaveric donor.)

Posttransplant survival world-wide from cadaveric donor single lung transplantation is 71% at one year and 65% at two years.[25] Most patients experience at least one or two episodes of acute rejection in the first month posttransplant; therefore recipients of cadaveric lungs require extensive pre- and postoperative regimens of immunosuppressive therapy. Consequently, the risk of posttransplant bacterial, viral and fungal infection is high and is the most common cause of death posttransplant. Therefore, complex regimens of pre- and posttransplant prophylaxis have been developed.

Potential recipients of live donor lungs must be made aware that pre- and posttransplant drug and therapy regimens are arduous and that return to ambulatory activity, i.e. play, school, employment, is by no means assured. Chronic patienthood may deprive children of the social interaction and experience necessary for emotional growth and development.[26] Patients of any age often tire of the frequent hospital visits and the burden of the drug regimen and want to break free from the strict lifestyle.[27] At this time it is unclear to what extent, if any, the unknown risks related to LDLT may be greater than the previously described risks associated with receiving a cadaveric transplant. In fact, the risks related to LDLT may be less because patients can be transplanted before they become desperately ill on the waiting list and because the closer genetic match from a related donor, may in theory, reduce both the frequency of rejection episodes and the need for immunosuppression.

Compared to recipients of cadaveric lung grafts, however, patients receiving a transplant from a live donor may be disadvantaged because the operation is new and technical proficiency is likely to improve with experience. Also, only a lobe rather than a whole lung is transplanted. The long-term implications of the concomitant reduction in pulmonary capacity are not known. Recipients who are growing children face the additional risk of future pulmonary insufficiency if the transplanted lobe cannot meet the increased demands caused by growth. This risk is similar for children receiving a cadaveric lung transplant.

Benefits

With regard to the benefits of LDLT, for patients with end-stage pulmonary disease there is no alternative therapy. Transplantation remains their only hope. Therefore, if LDLT should prove successful the beneficiaries will be patients who otherwise would have died while waiting for a cadaveric lung donor. As noted above, 54 patients died in the U.S. on the waiting list for a lung in 1990. By increasing the donor pool the recipient pool may also be expanded enabling more patients to be considered for a transplant. The use of lungs from live donors means elimination of the stress associated with waiting for a suitable cadaveric lung which may come at any unanticipated time, or may not come at all. Lastly, it is conceivable that posttransplant survival will be enhanced by using live donor lungs because the

procedure can be scheduled electively, with minimum ischemic time for the organ, optimum pre-conditioning of the recipient, and a maximized HLA matching.[28]

DONORS

Harms

The donor faces the risk of lobectomy which can be estimated from the 30-day surgical mortality rate for lobectomy in patients with lung cancer, which is <2% for patients under age 60.[29] However, mortality is likely to be less for lung donors because they would likely be free of any pulmonary or systemic disease.[30] While every effort can be made to minimize risk to the donor, perioperative and long-term complications are not negligible.[31] There are the usual perioperative risks of anesthetic mishaps, drug reactions, aspiration pneumonia, pulmonary emboli, myocardial infarction and so on. There may also be long-term compromise to pulmonary function associated with the reduced pulmonary reserve. Of course, donors will experience the ordinary postoperative discomforts that usually follow thoracotomy and general anesthesia.

Negative psychological sequelae from donating may be exacerbated when the donor feels pressured into donating or when the recipient has a bad outcome or dies. In addition, a donor may become depressed following the loss of an organ or because of newly created family conflicts.[32] Changes in family dynamics and structure are inevitable after live related donor transplantation with children but these changes need not be negative.[33] In fact there may be a strengthening of the family unit and a sense of investment in the child which is stronger than in cadaveric organ recipient families.[34]

Benefits

The main benefit to the donor is psychological — that is, knowing that one has attempted to save the life of the recipient, typically a loved one.[35] Even if the transplant is unsuccessful the attempt to reduce the suffering of a loved one may contribute to altruistic feelings and improved self-esteem which may persist.[36] These psychological benefits of donation will likely outweigh any negative psychosocial sequelae.[37]

IMPACT ON THE HEALTH CARE SYSTEM

In addition to the impact on recipients and donors, LDLT may provide benefits to hospitals and the health care system. An increased supply of lungs for transplant, available on an elective basis, may result in improved utilization of many resources including Intensive Care Units and Operating Rooms. Blood usage may be reduced through using autologous blood donation by the donor and donor-directed blood transfusions for the recipient. There may be a reduction in donor-related transplant costs. Lastly, due to the improved health of the recipient prior to transplantation and the excellent quality of the graft, there is likely to be a reduction in posttransplant costs.

CONSENT

The Belmont Report states that the ethical principle of respect for persons requires investigators to acknowledge the autonomy of each potential subject and to protect those subjects with diminished autonomy.[17] Respect for persons is the principle that underlies the need for, and the doctrine of, informed consent. The informed consent process involves disclosure of information by an investigator, a competent person's comprehension of the information and voluntary decision to proceed.[38] In this section we will examine the issue of consent as it pertains to LDLT.

RECIPIENTS

A clinical investigator has an obligation to fully disclose all information necessary for a potential subject's considered decision.[17] In LDLT this disclosure should include a clear explanation of the procedure's novel and unproven nature, the results thus far in the small number of procedures done, the mechanics of the surgery, the anticipated perioperative risks, the potential long-term risks and the requirement for life-long follow-up and compliance with the therapy and drug regimen.

If the potential subject is an adult, that individual's autonomous decision to proceed or not is sufficient. However, LDLT may most often find application in children. Children are presumed to be incompetent to consent to medical treatment and, therefore, proxy consent is necessary. The goal of proxy consent is to ensure that an individual's prior wishes are carried out or, if the prior wishes are not known, to act in the best interest of the individual. In the case of a child, who has never been competent, his or her prior wishes are unknown and so the parent will give proxy consent for the child according to the child's best interest. A potential problem arises since the parent who gives proxy consent may also be the donor of the lung graft. However, since no parent is likely to accept the risk of being a donor if he or she believes the LDLT procedure is not in the child's best interest, the fact that a parent is willing to donate may actually validate the goal of the proxy consent.

DONORS

Since there is no physical benefit from the donor lobectomy, great attention must be paid to the voluntariness of the donor's decision. The autonomy of potential donors is an important ethical concern in LDLT. In LDLT, donor consent which is truly voluntary may be a laudable but elusive goal. When a loved one's life hangs in the balance and a cadaver organ is not available, can consent be truly voluntary? Feelings of guilt over reluctance to donate and fear of criticism or rejection by other family members are important additional factors to consider in determining whether the consent process is truly voluntary.

Potential donors who are parents of potential recipients will inevitably feel considerable internal pressure to donate because without the transplant the child will likely get sicker and die. The extent of this internal pressure will increase with the severity of the child's illness. A 'cooling off period', that is a period of time between consenting for donation and the actual procedure, would enable potential donors to sort through their feelings regarding donations and give them time to seek counselling to address the internal pressure. In this context, psychiatric consultation may help to protect the right of the potential donor to refuse without guilt.[39]

Another way to address the problem of internal pressure would be to select potential recipients who are not critically ill. A noncritical case which requires less urgent attention generates less internal pressure on the potential donor and makes the cooling off period a possibility. This approach clearly would result in a better quality informed consent but it is not clear that it would be ethically more acceptable because thus far the standard lung transplant seems to have a more favorable outcome than the LDLT.

External pressure to donate may be exerted by the health care team or even other family members. Maintaining confidentiality in discussions with potential donors may enable them to refuse to become donors without facing pressure from others. If physicians keep the reasons for noneligibility confidential, especially when refusal is the reason, the extent of potential external pressure to donate will be reduced.

When disclosing information about LDLT, clinical investigators must be careful not to tailor the disclosure in such a way as to exert external pressure on the potential donor. The probability and magnitude of all potential harms, short- and long-term, associated with the lobectomy should be disclosed and the potential donor's questions should be answered. The assistance of a third-party as 'consent advocate'[20] may help to ensure that information is disclosed fully and fairly.

A psychiatric consultation may also be necessary to ensure that the potential donor can give a consent which is free from external coercion, and further, is mentally fit to undergo the rigors of donation. In this case, the duty of the consultant is to the best interest of the potential donor, not the best interest of the potential recipient nor the best interest of the medical team. This may create tensions between the heath care workers, the parents and the consultant. To avert any problems, the role of the psychiatric consultant must be made clear to all from the outset.[39]

SUBJECT SELECTION

The Belmont principle of justice demands the fair distribution of benefits and burdens in research which affects the selection of subjects.[17] This is difficult in LDLT because the primary benefit is to the recipient and the primary burden is to the donor. However, in this section we will examine the selection of subjects for LDLT.

RECIPIENTS

Since the principal benefit of LDLT is an increased chance of survival for those recipients who would have died while on the waiting list, potential recipients should not be selected from those who can survive on a waiting list for a lengthy period of time. Patients who are 'too well' can survive while awaiting a suitable cadaveric lung. Likewise, selecting the sickest patients (the 'desperate case' scenario[40,41]) will not ensure that potential benefit is maximized because such critically ill patients are likely to die even with a transplant. Patients should be selected who are not critically ill, but who are deteriorating clinically and are unlikely to survive for an extended time while waiting on a list for a cadaveric donor lung. These patients would benefit most from LDLT. Therefore, it is necessary for experienced clinicians to evaluate each patient on a case-by-case basis to determine who will most likely benefit from LDLT. An additional justification for this selection criterion is that maximizing potential recipient benefit also maximizes potential psychological benefit for donors. Also, it means the probability of harm to the donor exists in relation to a more probable good outcome for the recipient.

Selecting patients who are not critically ill also alleviates the pressure on potential donors to consent in an emergency situation when pressure is at its maximum. As noted, allowing potential donors time to consider the potential harms and benefits of donating is a procedural means for helping to ensure a substantively sound consent.

DONORS

Donors may be related to the recipient in two ways. They may be genetically related, such as a parent, sibling or child; or they may be emotionally related, such as a spouse or friend. In order to maximize benefit to the recipient, genetically related individuals should be selected as potential donors. In order to maximize benefit to the donor, that is psychological benefit, emotionally related individuals should be selected as donors. Therefore, when the potential donor is both genetically and emotionally related to the recipient, potential benefit is maximized. In the majority of cases of LDLT a parent will be the most appropriate donor for his or her child.

It is harder to justify selecting a potential donor who is genetically related but emotionally unrelated to the recipient, such as an absentee parent or an estranged sibling, or one who is emotionally related but genetically unrelated, such as a spouse, step-parent or close friend. These individuals may be selected as potential donors in the future but only after the probability of recipient benefit has been established and the motivations of the potential donor have been carefully scrutinized.

Individuals who are both genetically and emotionally unrelated to the recipient, despite being less predisposed to coercion or pressure, are less likely to contribute to maximizing the benefits of LDLT and should not be selected at this time.

THE ROLE OF THE IRB

The task of an Institutional Review Board (IRB) is to ensure that proposed research meets legal and ethical standards in order to protect the interest of potential subjects. IRBs evaluate the methods of obtaining informed consent, the potential harms and benefits, and the selection of subjects. In this section we will discuss the way in which an IRB can or cannot determine the ethical acceptability of the potential harms and benefits of LDLT.

The Belmont Report states:

It is commonly said that benefits and risks must be "balanced" and shown to be "in a favorable ratio." The metaphorical character of these terms draws attention to the difficulty of making precise judgments. Only on rare occasions will quantitative techniques be available for the scrutiny of research protocols. However, the idea of systematic, nonarbitrary analysis of risks and benefits should be emulated insofar as possible.[17]

The problem with this proposal, for an IRB, is that potential harms and benefits lack a basis of comparison—they are incommensurable. There are two types of incommensurability, both of which are relevant to LDLT. First, harms and benefits may affect different domains of health status. For example, a subject may incur a physical risk in expectation of a potential psychological benefit. Second, harms and benefits may affect different people. In LDLT, the principal risk is assumed by the donor but the principal benefit accrues to the recipient. Moreover, donors assume a physical risk but potentially gain a psychological benefit. The harms and benefits are of different types with no common measurement and are distributed between different people. Therefore, they are incommensurable.

In the face of this incommensurability, how are the potential harms and benefits of LDLT to be evaluated? Only individuals can know how different incommensurable influences affect them personally. The personal subjective understanding of the way in which harms and benefits can affect an individual is the common scale which allows the prospective subject to 'weigh the risks and benefits' to determine the acceptability of the balance. In LDLT, only the competent potential recipients and donors, or, in the case of a child who is a potential recipient, the potential donor-parent, can determine whether the potential harms are acceptable in light of the potential benefits.

Clearly, an IRB cannot do what it is expected to do which is to 'weigh risks and benefits' or evaluate the 'risk/benefit ratio.' Even after clarifying the distinction between risk and harm, for an IRB, potential harms and benefits are incommensurable. We will now propose a revision of the role of the IRB which will offer a procedural means for avoiding the evaluation of incommensurables in research protocols.

We suggest that the IRB should determine whether LDLT is an acceptable research endeavor for its particular institution. Assistance from the institution's mission statement may be helpful in this regard. A mission statement is developed by an institution's Board of Directors and defines the "purpose, philosophy, values, and services of a health care facility."[42] It may also articulate a commitment to 'quality of care', areas of expertise, or delineate morally acceptable and unacceptable actions within the institution.[43] In an institution where medical research takes place, the institution's mission statement should also specify the type of research that is acceptable in that institution. This will be determined by practical factors such as resources, facilities and personnel, but also by moral factors such as purpose, philosophy and values. Dr. Frances Moore suggested three points to consider in such a determination: 1) the scientific background of the procedure; 2) the field strength of the team; and 3) the ethical climate of the institution.[41] The acceptability of types and magnitudes of harm is not determined empirically by probabilities or outcome measures, but by community values. This subjective determination of acceptable risk in research is a moral activity which should be undertaken by those accountable to the community—the Board of Directors.

The role then of the IRB should be to determine whether LDLT is acceptable research at the institution, and if so, to work with the investigators to ensure that the protocol maximizes the potential for benefit and minimizes the potential for harm, and gives potential subjects all information material to their decision regarding consent. The IRB must also assure that the consent process is as clear and noncoercive as possible. Then potential recipients and donors can decide for themselves whether the risks and benefits are in acceptable balance. (It should be noted that this proposed role of the IRB in the case of LDLT is not the current role of the IRB under federal law.)

RESEARCH ETHICS CONSULTATION

Research ethics consultation is another means for ensuring the ethical acceptability of research protocols. Before the implementation of an innovative therapy, discussions between investigators and clinical ethicists may be helpful in identifying and addressing the key ethical issues which are raised by the innovation. Seminars open to a hospital or university community can also add to the ethical forethought. The result of this consultation may then serve as the basis for the proposal to be submitted to the IRB. With the ethical issues addressed proactively, greater attention can then be directed toward implementation. The feasibility and potential advantage of this method has been demonstrated in live donor liver transplantation.[20,21]

CONCLUSION

Live donor lung transplantation may become an acceptable alternative for patients suffering from end-stage pulmonary disease. It may be particularly beneficial for those patients who would likely die on a waiting list for a transplantable cadaveric lung. However, LDLT is a novel and unvalidated practice. We recommend that it only be undertaken within the context of a research protocol which is designed to maximize the potential benefits to recipients and minimize the risks. There are several ethical concerns that must be considered when implementing a protocol for LDLT. These concerns are both substantive and procedural and pertain to the types of potential harms and benefits, consent, and recipient and donor selection. We recommend that consent be obtained over a period of time, that potential recipients be clinically deteriorating but not critically ill, and that potential donors should be both genetically and emotionally related to the potential recipient. If pursued with scientific and ethical rigor, LDLT may someday prove to be a medically beneficial treatment for hopelessly ill patients while at the same time becoming a source of emotional satisfaction for donors who have done what they could to save their loved one.

References

1. Theodore J, Lewiston N. Lung transplantation comes of age. N Engl J Med 1990; 322:772-4.
2. Morrison DL, Maurer JR, Grossman RF. Preoperative assessment for lung transplantation. Clinics in Chest Medicine 1990; 11:207-15.
3. UNOS Update, May 1992; 8:2.
4. UNOS Update, October 1992; 8:47.
5. UNOS Update, January 1992; 8:18.
6. UNOS Update, January 1991; 7:23.
7. UNOS Update, July 1992; 8:37.
8. UNOS Update, June 1992; 8:14,16.
9. Kolata G. Lungs from parents fail to save girl, 9, and doctors assess ethics. New York Times, May 20, 1991:A11.
10. Levine RJ. Ethics and regulation of clinical research. 2nd ed. New Haven: Yale University Press, 1988:3-7.
11. Levine RJ. Clarifying the concepts of research ethics. Hastings Center Report 1979; 9:21-6.
12. Medical Research Council of Canada, Guidelines for Research Involving Human Subjects. (Ottawa: Minister of Supply and Services Canada), 1987:19.
13. Jonsen AR, Siegler M, Winslade WJ.

Clinical ethics. 3rd ed. New York: McGraw-Hill, Inc., 1992:147.
14. "The Nuremberg Code". In Annas GJ, Grodin MA, eds. The Nazi Doctors and the Nuremberg Code. New York: Oxford University Press, 1992:2.
15. World Medical Association. Declaration of Helsinki IV. 41st World Medical Assembly, Hong Kong, September 1989. Reprinted in Annas GJ and Grodin MA eds., The Nazi Doctors and the Nuremberg Code. New York: Oxford University Press, 1992; Appendix 3:339-42.
16. The Council for International Organizations of Medical Sciences. International Guidelines for Ethical Review of Epidemiological Studies. Geneva: CIOMS, 1991.
17. U.S. National Commission for the Protection of Human Subjects of Biomedical and Behavioral Research. The Belmont Report: Ethical Principles and Guidelines for the Protection of Human Subjects of Research. Washington: Department of Health, Education and Welfare, 1979.
18. Federal Register, Part II, Federal Policy for the protection of Human Subjects; Notices and Rules, 1991; Vol. 56, No. 117: s. 111.
19. Singer PA, Siegler M, Whitington PF et al. Equipoise and the ethics of segmental liver transplantation. Clin Res 1988; 36:539-45.
20. Singer PA, Siegler M, Whitington PF et al. Ethics of liver transplantation with living donors. N Engl J Med 1989; 321:620-2.
21. Singer PA, Siegler M, Lantos JD et al. The ethical assessment of innovative therapies: liver transplantation with living donors. Theore Med 1990; 11:87-94.
22. Shaw LR, Miller JD, Slutsky AS et al. Ethics of lung transplantation with live donors. Lancet 1991; 338:678-81.
23. Federal Register, Part II. Federal policy for the protection of human subjects; notices and rules. 1991; 56(117):s. 111(a)(2).
24. World Medical Association. Declaration of Helsinki IV. 41st World Medical Assembly, Hong Kong, September 1989. Reprinted in Annas GJ and Grodin MA eds, The Nazi Doctors and the Nuremberg Code. New York: Oxford University Press, 1992;

Appendix 3:339-42.

25. Miller JD, Ramirez J, deHoyos A, Patterson A. Isolated lung transplantation. Can J Surg 1992; 35:351-7.

26. Scharschmidt BF. Human liver transplantation: analysis of data on 540 patients from four centers. Hepatology 1984; 4:95s-101s.

27. Caplan AL, Annas G, Bazell R, Burrows L, Miller C, Swazey J. The gift of life: dilemmas in organ transplantation. Mount Sinai Journal of Medicine 1989; 56:395-405.

28. Riehle RA, Steckler R, Naslkund EB. Selection criteria for the evaluation of living related renal donors. J Urol 1990; 144:845-8.

29. Ginsberg RJ, Hill LD, Eagan RT et al. Modern thirty-day operative mortality for surgical resection in lung cancer. J Thorac Cardiovasc Surg 1983; 86:654-8.

30. Deslauriers J, Ginsberg RJ, Dubois P et al. Current operative morbidity associated with elective surgical resection for lung cancer. Can J Surg 1989; 5:335-9.

31. Dunn JF, Nylander WA Jr., Richie RE et al. Living related kidney donors: a 14 year experience. Ann Surg 1986; 203:637-43.

32. Youngner S. Organ donation and procurement. In Craven J and Rodin G (eds.), Psychiatric Aspects of Organ Transplantation. Oxford: Oxford University Press, 1992.

33. Wiley FM, Lindamood MM, Pfefferbaum-Levine B. Donor-patient relationship in pediatric bone marrow transplantation. J Assoc Pediatric Oncology Nurses 1984; 1:8-14.

34. Whitington PF, Siegler M, Broelsch CE. Living donor nonrenal organ transplantation: a focus on living related orthotopic liver transplantation, in Land W, and Dossetor JB (eds.) Organ Replacement Therapy: Ethics, Justice and Commerce.

Berlin: Springer Verlag, 1991; p.125.

35. Stiller CR, Lindberg MC, Rimstead D et al. Living related donation. Transplant Proc 1985; XVII(Suppl 3):85-100.

36. Fellner CH, Marshal JR. Kidney donors - the myth of informed consent. Am J Psychiatry 1970; 126:79-85.

37. Simmons RG. Psychological reactions to giving a kidney, in Levy NB (ed), Psychonephrology 1: psychological factors in hemodialysis and transplantation. New York: Plenum, 1981.

38. President's Commission for the Study of Ethical Problems in Medicine and Biomedical and Behavioral Research, Making Health Care Decisions: the Ethical and Legal Implications of Informed Consent in the Patient-Practitioner Relationship, Volume I. Washington: U.S. Government Printing Office, 1982.

39. Lowy FH, Martin DK. Ethical considerations in transplantation. In: Craven J and Rodin GM eds. Psychiatric Aspects of Organ Transplantation, Oxford: Oxford University Press, 1992.

40. Moore FD. The desperate case: CARE (Cost, Applicability, Research, Ethics). JAMA 1989; 261:1483-4.

41. Moore FD. Three ethical revolutions: ancient assumptions remodelled under pressure of transplantation. Transplant Proc 1988; XX(suppl 1):1061-7.

42. Reeves PN. Strategic planning for hospitals. Chicago: American College of Hospital Administrators, 1983.

43. Miles SH, Singer PA, Siegler M. Conflicts between patients' wishes to forgo treatment and the policies of health care facilities. N Engl J Med 1989; 321:48-50.

INDEX

Items in italics denote figures (*f*) or tables (*t*).